CW00819136

Jan Swanson, D.O.
Alan Cooper, Ph.D.

Relapse and HIV Risk

HAZELDEN

Hazelden
Center City, Minnesota 55012-0176

About the pamphlet. Whether we know or have heard of
someone with it, HIV affects all of us. HIV and its related
problems pose a big risk for relapse. This pamphlet will give
you practical information about HIV and AIDS. It will teach
you how to cope and give you other facts and skills you need,
even if you are not HIV-positive.

Some of the material in **The Complete Relapse Prevention
Skills Program** *is adapted from Marlatt's Model of Relapse
Prevention as published in the book* **Relapse Prevention.**
*Diagrams of the model and quotes from the book are used
with the permission of G. Alan Marlatt and Guilford Press.*

The Complete Relapse Prevention Skills Program
is dedicated to our fathers, Walt and Paul, who would
have enjoyed seeing it in print.

—Jan Swanson
Alan Cooper

ACKNOWLEDGMENTS

We recognize Alan Marlatt, Ph.D., and Judith Gordon, Ph.D.; their research efforts are the foundation of our program. We thank Juan Martinez, Laura Albrecht, R.N., C.A.D.A.C., Larry Stone, R.N., and Ed Dolgorukov, J.D., for their thoughtful suggestions and advice; DeeDee Harris, Chellie Bowden, and Carole Wood for their help in typing the manuscript; Tom Jones for his administrative support and encouragement; and last, but not least, we thank our editors Judy Delaney, Sid Farrar, and Don Freeman for their thoughtful editing and for believing in us. A special thanks to Doug Toft for his hard work on this program.

We welcome your comments. You can write us at:

Jan Swanson, D.O., and Alan Cooper, Ph.D.
1244 South Ridge Court, Suite 103
Hurst, Texas 76053

INTRODUCTION

G. Alan Marlatt
Addictive Behaviors Research Center
University of Washington
Seattle, Washington

WHEN I FIRST STARTED WORKING AS A PSYCHOLOGIST in the addiction treatment field more than twenty-five years ago, relapse was a taboo topic. In those days, relapse was equated with failure, and abstinence or sobriety was equated with success, a strict dichotomy that left no middle ground. Although everyone knew cases of successful recovery from addiction, treatment outcome studies continued to show high relapse rates. Relapse was viewed as a negative outcome, a dead end on the road to recovery.

Then things began to change. Relapse began to be studied as a process over time, not just a fixed, negative outcome. We started to realize that people recover at different rates. Many who achieved an eventual stable recovery reported that they had passed over a rocky road of relapse on their way to sobriety. Others managed to recover without a lapse. Some people found help in Twelve Step support groups while others sought other forms of help or struggled on their own. Research revealed that many roads can lead to eventual recovery, a finding that has led to today's emphasis on matching specific treatment methods to each particular individual's strengths and needs.

Much of what we have learned about relapse prevention has come directly from the stories and accounts people in recovery have given us. Comparing people who were successful treatment "survivors" with those who were more prone to relapse revealed a number of practical coping methods and strategies that could be helpful if passed on to those in the early stages of treatment and recovery. The good news about relapse is that one can learn to prevent it. Or, should relapse occur, a variety of coping methods are available to help one get back on track as soon as possible. For many, relapse is an essential part of the recovery process; the more we understand it, the better we can handle it if it occurs.

Just as relapse can be considered a process, recovery itself can be thought of as a journey, a journey you do not have to make entirely on your own.

The relapse prevention materials developed by Dr. Swanson and Dr. Cooper are designed to help you on the journey of recovery, and I recommend them highly. Think of them as a combination driver's guide and maintenance manual for the trip ahead. Bon voyage!

PREVIEW

All of us are living with HIV, whether we want to or not. Many of us know of someone—a celebrity, friend, or family member—who has been diagnosed as HIV-positive or who has AIDS.

HIV disease especially affects recovering people. Even if you are not HIV-positive, you probably know someone in recovery who is. You may know someone who has died of AIDS. Many of us had unsafe sex while drunk or high. Others shared needles with other drug users. Such actions put us at risk for HIV infection.

If you want to stay sober and clean, learn how

HIV affects you. This is a big assignment. Think of handling it in two stages. In stage one, see HIV infection as a personal risk, take a close look at your sexual behavior, and commit yourself to staying sober. During stage two, think about getting tested for HIV infection. Learn to handle this situation so that you do not relapse.

Also remember that being diagnosed as HIV-positive or getting AIDS can be a great challenge to your sobriety. How you cope with such facts will make a big difference to your recovery and to your good health.

Many recovering people relapse when faced with HIV disease because they lack coping skills. This pamphlet is about gaining the facts and skills you need—even if you are not HIV-positive. You'll read about the following topics:

Stage one: Seeing HIV infection as a personal risk

☐ Learn about HIV and AIDS
☐ Practice safer sex
☐ Commit yourself to staying sober

Stage two: Deciding about HIV testing

☐ Marty's story
☐ Linda's story
☐ Coping skills—the crucial difference
☐ Consider your personal risk for HIV infection
☐ Learn about HIV testing
☐ Deal with shame and anxiety
☐ Choose a place and time to test
☐ Plan to prevent relapse

STAGE ONE:
SEEING HIV INFECTION AS A PERSONAL RISK

John was a thirty-five-year old businessman. He was recovering from addiction to prescription drugs. Since he dated only professional women, he never bothered with condoms. "These women are too smart and too classy to be HIV-positive," John said. "And anyway, only homosexuals get AIDS. I'm not at any risk."

John's sponsor disagreed. "Your behavior is self-destructive," he told John. "Your partner can be HIV-positive, even if she doesn't look sick. HIV can affect all women—even the 'classy' ones."

After John learned more about HIV, he decided that his sexual behavior was unsafe. By learning to practice safer sex, he reduced his risk of HIV infection and relapse as well.

Learn about HIV and AIDS. Like John, you can start by learning some basic facts about HIV. Knowing these facts is a first step to protecting yourself.

Begin with the answers to these seven questions:

(1) What does *HIV* stand for?
(2) What are CD4 cells?
(3) What is a low CD4 count?
(4) What is AIDS?
(5) Are HIV and AIDS the same?
(6) How is HIV spread?
(7) If I get HIV disease or AIDS, will I die right away?

(1) *What does HIV stand for?* These letters stand
for *Human Immunodeficiency Virus*. To get a handle
on this term, break it down into smaller parts:

- ❐ HUMAN means only people get infected with
  HIV. Dogs, cats, and other animals do not.
- ❐ IMMUNO refers to your immune system. It con-
  sists of the organs and cells in your body that
  fight off infection.
- ❐ DEFICIENCY means that something is lacking.
  So, immunodeficiency means that the body is
  not killing off diseases or infections well.
- ❐ A VIRUS is a tiny organism that causes diseases. HIV is a virus that can enter your body's
  cells and prevent them from working to keep
  you healthy.

(2) *What are CD4 cells?* HIV especially affects
the CD4 cells, a type of blood cell. CD4 cells are little
warriors that kill off infections. HIV enters the CD4
cells and destroys them. As HIV disease progresses, a
person's CD4 cells fall in number. When that happens,
the person more easily gets infection and disease.

People with impaired immune systems can get
opportunistic infections. These take advantage of a
weakened immune system. They include:

- ❐ Pneumocystis Carinii Pneumonia (also
  called PCP)
- ❐ Mycobacterium Avium Complex (MAC), which
  causes life-threatening diarrhea
- ❐ Cytomegalovirus (CMV), which can invade the
  retina of the eyes and cause blindness

You are unlikely to catch these diseases unless your immune system is weakened. People with healthy immune systems rarely get opportunistic infections unless they have cancer or use certain drugs.

In short, HIV is like a foreign army. It invades and kills your little warriors—the CD4 cells—and leaves you open to attack from infections.

(3) *What is a low CD4 count?* Doctors can measure the number of CD4 cells in your blood. The figure they give you is a CD4 count—the number of CD4 cells in one cubic millimeter of blood. (A cubic millimeter of blood is about the size of a grain of sugar.) A person without HIV has between 500 and 1800 CD4 cells per cubic millimeter.

If you hear that someone has a low CD4 count, this could mean several things:

❐ When the CD4 count is between 200 and 500, the person's immune system is weakened a little. However, this person is not in great danger of getting an opportunistic infection. (Many people start taking antiviral medications at this point, however.)

❐ If the CD4 count is between 100 and 200, the immune system is much more depressed. At this stage people can get PCP, so it's important for them to take preventive medicine.

❐ When the CD4 count is less than 100, the immune system is weak. The risk for opportunistic infection is great. People at this stage must take medicine and see a physician. Even so, people with a CD4 count of less than 50 can still be healthy.

(4) *What is AIDS?* AIDS stands for *Acquired Immunodeficiency Syndrome:*

- ❒ ACQUIRED means that people are not born with the illness but get it later in life. By the way, infants are not "born" with AIDS; they *can* be born with HIV in their blood.
- ❒ IMMUNODEFICIENCY means that the immune system is damaged and cannot fight off many infections.
- ❒ SYNDROME means someone suffers from opportunistic infections.

(5) *Are HIV and AIDS the same?* HIV and AIDS are *not* the same thing. To understand this, keep the following points in mind:

- ❒ HIV is the virus that can lead to AIDS. Being HIV-positive does not mean that you have AIDS.
- ❒ You cannot "catch" AIDS, but you can get infected with HIV.
- ❒ You can have AIDS without appearing sick.

AIDS does develop at some point in most people who are HIV-positive, mainly because the Centers for Disease Control defines AIDS as a CD4 count of less than 200. But remember that you can have a low CD4 count and still be free from disease.

(6) *How is HIV spread?* HIV is spread by contact with blood, vaginal fluids, and semen. You can get HIV from having sex or by sharing needles with drug users. Pregnant women can also pass HIV on to their babies.

The following are *not* ways you can get HIV from people who are HIV-positive:

- ☐ sitting next to them
- ☐ hugging them or shaking hands
- ☐ eating food they've cooked
- ☐ sitting on a toilet seat they've used
- ☐ being close to them when they sneeze
- ☐ coming in contact with their sweat

Abusing alcohol or other drugs raises your risk of HIV infection. First, alcohol itself depresses your immune system. Each time you drink heavily, your immune system gets weaker. As a result, you are more likely to get infected with HIV and other diseases as well. What's more, using chemicals can impair your judgment. When you're high, you're more likely to practice unsafe sex or share needles.

HIV is not spread by "high-risk groups." It is spread when people *act* in high-risk ways. Your behavior determines your risk for HIV infection.

Don't be afraid of people who are HIV-positive. They need your support, friendship, and occasional hugs.

(7) *If I get HIV disease or AIDS, will I die right away?* *HIV is not a death sentence.* Even if you develop AIDS, you can live for years. One London hospital did a follow-up study of 111 patients who were HIV-positive. The study found that death in HIV patients was rare before their CD4 count fell below 50. Many patients remained above 50 for twelve years after becoming HIV-positive. Amazingly, there was a better than 50-percent chance for patients to be alive even when their CD4 count was zero. These patients got regular medical care and took medicine to prevent infections. HIV patients should begin medical care early, as this extends their life.

Practice safer sex. Linda had not used alcohol for twelve months. While at a friend's house on New Year's Eve, she saw Jim, an old boyfriend. Linda was still attracted to Jim. She felt tempted to have sex with him. But she knew she'd feel comfortable with sex only if she had something to drink. When Jim came on to her for a kiss, she decided to leave the party.

Several weeks later, Jim told her that he was a hepatitis carrier and had AIDS. Linda was happy with her decision to abstain from, or not have, sex with Jim. Her story shows how to prevent sex from being a trigger for relapse or a way to spread HIV infection.

In the 1960s and 1970s, sex seemed easily available to many people—almost a harmless pastime. This is no longer true. Today, a one-night stand can be deadly. In New York, San Francisco, and other cities, AIDS is a leading killer. Other sexually transmitted diseases (STDs) infect thousands of young adults.

The AIDS and STD epidemics tell us something important: If we want to stay healthy, we must learn new skills before starting a sexual relationship. We must know how to prevent STDs such as HIV disease and AIDS.

Today, people are learning to practice safer sex. They're asking their partners to do the same. This is not easy, because it requires us to be honest about private matters. Recovering people would be wise to do the following before becoming sexually active:

Find out if you have an STD. *STD* is a term that applies to over twenty diseases. These diseases are spread when people exchange bodily fluids—semen, vaginal fluid, and blood. Pregnant women can also pass some STDs on to their infants. Among the STDs are chlamydia, genital herpes, gonorrhea, genital warts, syphilis, hepatitis, crabs, and hepatitis B.

To find out if you have an STD, get a complete physical exam. It should include blood work. Many people believe that they automatically got tested for STDs during alcohol or other drug treatment. Often this is *not* true. Find out for sure whether you've been tested.

If you are still in treatment, ask for a physical that includes lab tests for STDs. If your treatment center does not offer this service, ask for an appointment at your county health department.

Be sure to get tested to see if you have had hepatitis B. Ask about a hepatitis vaccine series. Hepatitis B can be fatal, but this vaccine will prevent your getting it.

You can learn more about STDs by calling the National STD Hot Line at 1-800-227-8922.

Talk to your partner about STDs. If you have HIV or another STD, tell your partner before you have sex. Always practice safer sex, and have sex only when your partner agrees to do the same.

Before having sex, find out if your partner has an STD or is at risk for HIV infection. You have a right to know. Remember, people with HIV or other STDs can look perfectly normal. They may not even *know* they have an STD.

Know which sexual activities are safer. When you practice safer sex, you have many options besides sexual intercourse. These include writing love letters, hugging, caressing, fondling, cuddling, massaging, dry kissing, and having "phone sex." If you have intercourse, use latex barriers—condoms or dental dams.

To prevent STDs, *avoid* the following activities. They are unsafe, high-risk behaviors.

- ❐ having intercourse (penetration) without a condom or dental dam
- ❐ sharing sex toys such as dildos and vibrators that have not been cleaned (Be sure to unplug sex toys and then clean them with bleach and soapy water.)
- ❐ having contact with blood, semen, or vaginal fluid
- ❐ sharing razors or toothbrushes

Before you start a sexual relationship, get tested for STDs, including HIV. Ask your partner to do the same. Before you stop using latex barriers, wait at least six months and get tested for HIV again. It takes that long to be reasonably sure you're safe.

In the meantime, practice safer sex. Remember that even intercourse using a condom or dental dam can still be risky.

Use a condom. Condoms are one type of latex barrier used to prevent HIV infection and other STDs. To reduce your risk of infection, use condoms with the following tips in mind. (These instructions are directed to men, but women should know them too.)

❐ *Always keep condoms on hand.* Store them in a cool, dry place that's away from sunlight. Special heavy-duty condoms are available. Using them is a good idea if you have anal intercourse.

❐ *Use latex condoms.* Sheepskin condoms allow you to pass HIV or germs on to your partner.

❐ *Never use a condom from a damaged package.* Never use a condom that is yellow, brittle, sticky, or shows other signs of aging or damage.

❐ *Use condoms only once.* Never reuse a condom.

❐ *Put the condom on your penis as soon as you have an erection.* Don't wait until you're ready to ejaculate. Do this before your penis touches your partner's vagina, anus, or mouth. The clear fluid that comes from your penis before you ejaculate can contain HIV and other germs that cause STDs.

❐ *After you put the condom on, you may want to use a lubricant.* If you are having anal intercourse, definitely use a lubricant. The anal opening is smaller and drier. It does not stretch as well as the vaginal opening. Using more lubricant will make the condom and the anus less likely to tear.

❐ *Never use oil-based lubricants such as Crisco, baby oil, hand lotion, Vaseline, massage oils, or whipped cream.* These can cause the condom to dissolve. Use only water-based lubricants like K-Y jelly. Condoms with Nonoxynol-9 are a good choice.

❏ *If you feel the condom coming off, hold it at the rim to keep it on.* If the condom does come off, put on a new one immediately—before you continue with sex.

❏ *When you decide to stop intercourse, hold the rim of the condom at the base of the penis as you withdraw.* Hold the condom in place as you withdraw.

❏ *Withdraw when your penis is still hard.* If it is soft, you will be more likely to spill semen on your partner.

❏ *If the condom breaks, pull out your penis immediately.* Remove the condom and wash your penis, genital area, and hands with soap and water. If you've had vaginal intercourse, your partner should put spermicide in her vagina right away.

❏ *If you and your partner are both HIV-positive, use condoms until you are both tested and examined for STDs.* Keep using condoms until you're found free of STDs. Remember that genital warts, herpes, and hepatitis B are very harmful to HIV-positive people. If you don't have these diseases now, you certainly don't want to catch them. Some experts believe you should continue to use condoms in any case. This is because you can get infected with a more dangerous strain of HIV than you have already.

Use a dental dam. If you don't know what a dental dam is, you're not alone. Most people don't know what they are, let alone how to use one.

You may have seen a dental dam in your dentist's office. The dam is a stretchy piece of latex that the dentist uses to keep your mouth sterile. In other words, it is a thin sheet of plastic used to cover an area in order to avoid direct contact with body fluids.

Use a dental dam if you plan on having mouth-to-vagina or mouth-to-anus sex. Apply the dental dam with a water-based lubricant to the vaginal opening or anus. This will help to prevent the spread of infection. You can get dental dams from your dentist or medical supply store. You can use plastic wrap from the kitchen or cut the tip off of a non-lubricated latex condom and then cut down the length of the condom to make your own sheet of plastic, which will provide the same function as a dental dam.

However, remember that *no* material or device has been tested and approved for safe oral sex. When it comes to spreading HIV disease and other STDs, oral sex is a high-risk behavior.

Commit yourself to staying sober. One important way to decrease your risk of HIV infection is to stay sober. Renew your commitment to sobriety in any way that works for you. One option is going to support groups such as Narcotics Anonymous or Alcoholics Anonymous. Another is putting your commitment in writing and posting it in a place where you'll see it often.

Perhaps you've tested negative for HIV, even though you've had unsafe sex or used needles to inject drugs. If so, commit yourself right now to staying clean and sober. Even though you've been fortunate so far, you are still at risk for HIV. When you stay sober, you're more likely to make good judgments about having sex and preventing HIV infection.

STAGE TWO:
DECIDING ABOUT HIV TESTING

Marty's story. Marty was a gay man, thirty-five years old. He was recovering from cocaine addiction. Before joining NA, Marty had often been high on cocaine while having sex. He'd forgotten who many of his partners were, let alone whether they practiced safer sex.

Now Marty often felt depressed and hopeless about HIV disease. He believed that his drug history and years of unsafe sex doomed him to being HIV-positive. Whenever he felt that way, he craved cocaine to lift his spirits.

One night, when the cravings were unusually strong, Marty called Julio, his sponsor in NA. Julio told Marty to get tested for HIV right away. According to Julio, fear of HIV infection put Marty at serious risk for relapse.

Marty agreed to be tested. Much to his surprise, the test was negative. He did not have HIV infection. With these results in hand, Marty decided to renew his commitment to sobriety and safer sex.

Linda's story. Linda was a thirty-eight-year-old woman who owned her own business. She'd been in recovery for eighteen months. Before getting drug treatment, she'd been a cocaine user and a heavy drinker of alcohol. She'd also traded sex for drugs.

When Linda was in treatment, she tested negative for HIV. She was overjoyed with the results. She planned to repeat the test six months later.

Shortly after leaving treatment, though, Linda found out that one of her former dealers had died of AIDS. At one time, Linda and this man had shared needles. When she learned of his death, Linda grew anxious. She knew she should test again for HIV but was terrified to do so.

Linda became so anxious that she thought of drinking again. She thought of finding a physician to prescribe her some tranquilizers. During her first month out of treatment, she relapsed.

Coping skills—the crucial difference. Both Marty and Linda had fears about HIV infection. Yet they responded to the fear in different ways. By calling his sponsor, Marty used an important coping skill to deal with cravings. In deciding to test, he acted with courage.

Linda lacked such skills. Instead of asking for support, she tried to drown her fears by using chemicals.

When they lack coping skills, people often find that testing for HIV infection, waiting for the results, and *getting* the results can be overwhelming triggers for relapse. Sometimes people who are afraid of testing say to themselves, "What's the point? If I'm HIV-positive, I'll just die anyway."

This is not good reasoning. For one thing, HIV infection is not a death sentence. The sooner you're tested, the sooner you can get medical care. That increases your chances for being healthy and living longer. If you do not get treated, HIV disease could progress faster. You could get life-threatening diseases sooner.

Remember, HIV is not spread by high-risk *groups,* but by high-risk *behavior.* It's not who you are that counts but what you *do.* If you are free of HIV right now, you have the power to *stay* free. And if you are HIV-positive, you can avoid infecting others.

So far, this pamphlet has been about seeing HIV as a personal issue, practicing safer sex, and committing yourself to recovery. By taking these actions, you lay a great foundation for staying sober in the face of HIV. Now take your skills to a new level. Learn how to make a sound decision about testing for HIV.

Consider your personal risk for HIV infection. Get tested for HIV if any of the following statements are true for you:

 ☐ *You shared needles during drug use.* Sharing needles puts blood that might be infected with HIV directly into your bloodstream. Sharing needles with someone who's infected with HIV is like giving yourself an "HIV shot." It's a sure way to become infected. Even if you haven't shared needles since 1977, you'd benefit from being tested. You could still be infected and not know it.

□ *You had unsafe anal sex with an infected person.* Anal sex tears the rectal skin. This could allow HIV into your bloodstream.

□ *You had unsafe vaginal sex with an infected person.* HIV can pass from your partner's body fluids into your own.

□ *You had unsafe oral sex with an infected person.* Your partner's body fluids can enter into your bloodstream through cuts in your mouth or gums. This is one way to spread HIV.

□ *You had sex with anyone who practiced at least one high-risk behavior.* These people are at risk for HIV infection.

□ *You had sex with people who have an STD.* You know these people have had unsafe sex. If they have one STD, they could easily have HIV disease also.

□ *You had unsafe sex with someone who's had many partners.* The more sexual partners people have, the higher their risk of HIV infection.

□ *You had blackouts from alcohol or other drugs.* Be sure to test for HIV infection if this has happened to you. Who knows what you may have done when in a chemical haze?

□ *You received a blood transfusion between 1977 and 1985, or you received blood products to treat hemophilia.* Some people were infected with HIV in these ways.

❏ *You have had unsafe sex with someone who you do not know well, and you do not know their drug use or sexual history.*

Learn about HIV testing. Finding out your HIV status actually involves two procedures: the ELISA test and the Western Blot test. There are other, more sensitive tests. They are not widely available.

The ELISA is a preliminary test; a Western Blot is needed to confirm the results of the ELISA. You must get positive results on *both* tests before you can say that you are HIV-positive. Many people who test positive on the ELISA do not have HIV infection. The Centers for Disease Control recommends that a person take the ELISA twice.

If you test positive on both the ELISA and the Western Blot, you'll go through some additional lab work. This includes a complete blood count, blood chemistries, a CD4 cell count, and tests for syphilis and hepatitis B.

If you are at risk for HIV infection, get tested at least every six months; do this for two years after stopping high-risk behaviors. It can take this long to be sure you are HIV-negative. Remember that between the time of infection and the time you test positive, there can be a gap of several months.

So far, no one can cure HIV infection. But with proper treatment, you can *manage* HIV infection. Being HIV-positive does not mean you have AIDS or that you will become seriously ill soon. Instead, being HIV-positive is like having diabetes or high blood pressure. With good medical care and sound health habits, you could live a productive life. Many people are still alive ten or more years after getting infected.

Deal with shame and anxiety. When testing, you may find it embarrassing to admit that you've acted in ways that put you at high risk for HIV infection. Perhaps these behaviors involved unsafe sex, multiple sex partners, sex with prostitutes, or sharing needles. If you're prone to shame, you may see such behaviors as "proof" that you're basically a worthless person. Such feelings can lead you to withdraw from other people so that no one will know about your past.

There is another option. You can hang on to your self-esteem. You can view chemical dependency as a disease that impaired your judgment. What's more, you are *not* your disease. Your judgment can improve now that you're sober.

To take responsibility for actions that harmed others, to make amends, and to learn from your mistakes is wise. At the same time, remember to look at yourself with compassion always. Admitting mistakes and making amends does *not* mean that you are a bad person. You are—like all of us—a fallible human being. At any point in your past, you did your best with what you knew at the time.

People avoid testing for a variety of reasons, especially when they have false beliefs such as *Finding out that you're HIV-positive is getting a death sentence* or *Even if you know your HIV status, there's nothing you can do to prevent getting AIDS.* Reading this pamphlet can help rid you of such errors.

Even so, you may still need help in reducing your
anxiety before you agree to be tested. Consider the
following suggestions:

- ❐ *Accept that you are anxious.* You did not choose
  to be anxious, and you cannot get rid of this
  feeling on command. Simply allow yourself to
  feel anxious.

- ❐ *Discuss your decision to test with a counselor or
  physician before you discuss this decision with
  your peers.* When you talk to peers first, you
  run the risk that they'll gossip or speculate
  about your health and past behavior. You may
  also experience unkind remarks or get false
  information about testing. Take advantage of a
  professional's promise to keep what you say
  confidential.

- ❐ *Practice deep breathing or another relaxation
  technique.* The workbook *Relapse and HIV Risk*
  includes instructions for such a technique. (See
  the accompanying workbook, pages 13-15.)

Choose a time and place to test. You can be
tested for HIV at your doctor's office, a clinic, or a public health center. For more ideas about where to test,
call the National AIDS Hot Line at 1-800-342-AIDS.
Deaf persons can call 1-800-243-7889. Those who
speak Spanish may want to call 1-800-344-7432.

Testing sites differ according to how they reveal
the test results. Some sites offer *anonymous testing:*
Instead of giving your name, you get a number. You

use this number to get your test results. Other sites offer *confidential testing:* You give your name, but you are the only person who can learn the results.

In any case, choose a site that offers good counseling before and after the test. This is especially important when testing triggers fear or anxiety. If possible, test on a day when you feel "up." Ask a friend to go with you.

Plan to prevent relapse. Maria's and Larry's story shows how to prevent testing from becoming a trigger for relapse.

As a recovering cocaine addict, Maria thought about her risk for HIV infection and decided to test. She chose a clinic run by volunteers where she could get counseling before and after testing.

Next, Maria set a date to test. Well before that time, she decided which friends and family members to ask for support. She also invited her sister and her minister to go with her to the test.

Maria then created a Circle of Support and posted it in her bedroom. The Circle of Support is a chart that listed Maria's sources of help, hope, and encouragement. In this chart, Maria included the names of family members, close friends, and support groups. She also included the titles of books, movies, and songs that she found inspiring. (You can learn more about this chart by using the pamphlet and workbook titled *Your Circle of Support.*)

After creating her circle, Maria wrote letters to people she could have infected with HIV. She held the letters for the moment, planning to send them only if she tested positive.

Finally the day for Maria's ELISA test arrived. During the test, Maria used a deep breathing technique to help herself relax. After the test was done, she went to an NA meeting.

When Maria went to the clinic to learn her test results, she was terrified. Even so, she used her relaxation skills and took her Circle of Support to the appointment. She was relieved to learn that she tested negative.

One of Maria's friends from NA, Larry, also decided to be tested. Larry had a long history of unsafe sex. He'd also shared needles with other addicts. For months he'd suspected that he was HIV-positive, even though he felt and looked healthy. He wanted to know whether his hunch was right. If it was, he planned to get medical treatment right away.

When Larry tested positive, he felt both afraid and relieved to discover the truth. He also thought that his decision to test showed courage. It was a change from his old habit of avoiding unpleasant tasks—something he often did when using drugs.

Larry told Maria about his test results. Immediately Maria became part of Larry's Circle of Support. In helping Larry, Maria also found a powerful reason to abstain from cocaine. She learned first-hand the meaning of a slogan she'd heard at an NA meeting: "It is in giving that we receive."

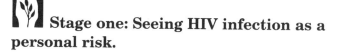 **Stage one: Seeing HIV infection as a personal risk.**

☐ *HIV stands for **Human Immunodeficiency Virus.*** This virus can affect the body's immune system—its ability to fight off disease.

☐ *HIV infection can lead to **AIDS** (**Acquired Immunodeficiency Syndrome**).* People with AIDS often get infections due to a weakened immune system.

☐ *HIV infection is not the same thing as AIDS.* Many people who are HIV-positive do not have AIDS. In fact, these people can be healthy and live for many years.

☐ *HIV is spread by contact with blood, vaginal fluid, and semen.* You can get HIV from having sex or from sharing needles. When giving birth, mothers can also pass HIV on to their children.

☐ *To prevent HIV infection, abstain from alcohol and other drugs.* Also, abstain from sex, or have sex only with uninfected people. During sex, avoid contact with blood, vaginal fluid, and semen. Use condoms and dental dams.

 Stage two: Deciding about HIV testing.

☐ *Review your personal history for behaviors that put you at risk for HIV infection.* Then decide whether to test.

▢ *If you **are** at risk for HIV infection, get tested at least every six months.* Do this for two years after stopping high-risk behaviors.

▢ *HIV testing actually involves two different lab procedures—the ELISA test and the Western Blot test.* You must test positive on both of them before you can say you're HIV-positive.

▢ *Forgive yourself for high-risk behaviors and plan to change them.* Also learn methods to relax and deal with anxiety.

▢ *If you decide to test for HIV, find a suitable place.* Also get counseling before and after testing.

▢ *Plan to prevent relapse during the testing process. Keep the following suggestions in mind:*

   ▢ *Decide who you can ask for emotional support.* Contact these people. Tell them that you are going to be tested. Ask if you can call or see them before and after your test. If possible, arrange for one of these people to come with you to the test.

   ▢ *Think about the people you've put at risk for HIV infection.* List their names. Decide how to contact them if you test positive. Before you test, write letters to these people; hold on to the letters until after you test. If you test positive, decide whether to send the letters. Don't send letters to people who could hurt you. Don't send the letters if doing so endangers your sobriety. Instead, ask the local health department to notify the people on your list without mentioning your name.

❐ *Plan to attend AA, NA, or another support group after you learn the results.* This is to remind you that sobriety comes first.

REFERENCES

American Social Health Association. *Positive Living*. Brochure written (1992) by the American Social Health Association, P.O. Box 13827, Research Triangle Park, NC 27709. (919) 361-8400.
Callen, Michael. *Surviving AIDS*. New York: HarperCollins, 1991.
Goldman, Lee. *HIV Disease - MKSAP-10*. Philadelphia: American College of Physicians, 1994.
McKay, Matthew, and Patrick Fanning. *Self-Esteem*. Oakland: New Harbinger Publications, 1987.
Moran, Fawn. *Taking Charge: A Planning Guide for People with HIV*. San Francisco: Impact AIDS, 1994.
Phillips, Andrew. "Immunodeficiency and the Risk of Death in HIV Infection." *Journal of the American Medical Association* 268, no. 19 (November 18, 1992):2662-6.
Schwartz, Ruth. *AIDS Medical Guide: A Series of Handbooks for People with HIV*. San Francisco: San Francisco AIDS Foundation, 1992.
Tilleraas, Perry. *Circle of Hope: Our Stories of AIDS, Addiction, and Recovery*. Center City, Minn.: Hazelden, 1990.
_____. *The Color of Light: Daily Meditations for All of Us Living with AIDS*. Center City, Minn.: Hazelden, 1988.

The relapse prevention materials developed by Dr. Swanson and Dr. Cooper are designed to help you on the journey of recovery, and I recommend them highly. Think of them as a combination Driver's Guide and Maintenance Manual for the trip ahead. Bon voyage!

-Dr. G. Alan Marlatt

The Complete Relapse Prevention Skills Program Part 2

This easily accessible program reinforces key relapse prevention concepts and fosters a client's confidence in their own coping abilities by identifying their strengths, building support, and increasing resiliency. Clients also learn to build on past successes and adopt new behaviors to maintain healthy sobriety.

Your Circle of Support

The information and exercises in *Your Circle of Support* help clients understand the importance of emotional and spiritual support, learn the positive qualities of sober, healthy friendships, and identify support resources.
Order No. 1627 Pamphlet, 32 pp.
Order No. 1626 Workbook, 28 pp.

Finding Your Strengths

This topic helps clients deal with self-criticism, develop new beliefs about themselves and others, and apply past relapse prevention successes to future high-risk situations.
Order No. 1629 Pamphlet, 32 pp.
Order No. 1628 Workbook, 32 pp.

Relapse and HIV Risk

Focusing on the connection between relapse and HIV risk, these materials provide clients with basic HIV information, including prevention of high-risk behaviors, testing procedures and resources, and tools to cope with either a positive or negative HIV test result.
Order No. 1624 Pamphlet, 32 pp.
Order No. 1623 Workbook, 28 pp.

For price and order information, or a free catalog, please call our Telephone Representatives.

Hazelden

Pleasant Valley Road • P.O. Box 176 • Center City, MN 55012-0176
1-800-328-9000 (Toll-Free, U.S., Canada & the Virgin Islands)
1-651-213-4000 (Outside the U.S. & Canada)
1-651-213-4590 (24-Hour FAX)
http://www.hazelden.org
Order No. 1624

ISBN 978-1-56838-905-9

DYING WORLD

MAGITECH LEGACY BOOK 1

CHRIS FOX

CHRIS FOX WRITES LLC

THE MAGITECH CHRONICLES

Buckle up, because you're about to enter *The Magitech Chronicles*. If you like *Dying World*, we have a complete seven-book prequel series with an ending already available.

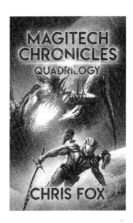

We're also working on a pen & paper RPG and the Kickstarter is going live right around the same time this book came out. You can learn more at magitechchronicles.com or our Magitech Chronicles World Anvil page.

We've got maps, lore, character sheets, and a free set of rules you can use to generate your own character.

I hope you enjoy!

-Chris

1

What would you risk for a chance at immortality? What dangers would you brave, if literal godhood were on the line? Most people will do damned near anything for a taste of that kind of power.

Our whole culture is built around lust for it. An entire planet of mercenaries, each clawing their way past the rest to get to the precious and infinitely rare magic, and the glory it brings.

Most won't admit, or don't even know, what that magic is. The tiny percentage who actually find the magic they seek are pillaging the corpses of gods. Deities who ruled this sector long before our ancestors came down out of the trees on whatever world gave us birth.

I can't ignore that fact. It's my job to understand those gods, and their ruins, and the battles they fought. That was the reason I was hired to come to this derelict deathtrap in the first place.

I'm an archeologist, though that isn't sexy enough for

today's holodrama crowd. They'd much prefer I call myself a relic hunter, which is an apt enough description, I guess.

I signed up to rob tombs, but found myself scavenging the dead hulks of ancient vessels long since picked clean by better men, and doing it alongside people who might not notice if my O_2 tank ran dry.

That was how I found myself in near darkness, prowling the claustrophobic air ducts aboard a colossus-class vessel constructed a hundred millennia ago. These ancient hulks orbit the extreme edges of the system, at the site of the barely remembered war that had marooned our people on the world of Kemet.

We'd come to pry whatever valuable parts or schematics still clung to her frigid bones, something that the people I'd signed on with were supposed to be very good at. They'd been at it for three years, if their spec-sheet was accurate, and were still flying, which seemed promising.

"Jerek, do you have a visual on the target?" A hard feminine voice crackled over the comm attached to my collar, causing me to jump.

That would be Sapphire. She was the hot one. I was still learning names, though Sapphire had warned me not to bother as I probably wouldn't survive. That was just hazing, or I hoped so anyway.

"If, uh, the target is the armory door, then yes," I whispered back as I shimmied to the edge of the duct. The grate was filled with triangular holes, just big enough to peer through at the blast door below. "Give me a minute to study it, and I'll confirm our intel."

"Is it the armory or not? And is it intact?" Sapphire hissed over the comm. "Just because we didn't see lurkers doesn't mean they aren't there. Why do you think they're called lurkers? They lurk. We need to get in, and get right back out again."

I didn't bother to answer, as I couldn't from my current location. The duct was above and to the side of the door, and I couldn't quite make out the runes along the rusty surface. They glowed with faint white-blue magic, the weak telltale remnant of a lingering enchantment just before it failed.

I paused to inspect the grate blocking my exit, which had no obvious fastenings. Of course, neither had the grate I'd entered through. The metal wasn't thick, but it was as strong as feathersteel, though a good deal heavier.

It had been built for utility, and not defense, thankfully. I reached for the holster attached to my flight suit along the right thigh, and withdrew my spellpistol.

Ariela, the name my father had given the sleek black weapon, was a fully developed eldimagus. A living magic item passed through our family for generations, maybe all the way back to planetfall. She could fire conventional rounds, sure. But she could also channel spells, if I supplied the magic.

I pressed the thick barrel against the corner of the grate, and caressed the trigger. The weapon instantly connected to me in a primal way well beyond sight, and tore a piece of *fire* magic from the reservoir in my chest. The magic built in the barrel for a split second, then a narrow beam of orange-white flame melted the metal into glowing rivulets even as the barrel of my weapon heated.

I repeated the process at each of the four corners, then holstered Ariela's still warm form. I wasn't looking forward to this next part, but at least no one was around to see me struggle.

It took several awkward moments to squirm around until my boots were planted against what remained of the grate. In an action holo it would have come loose on the first kick. Depths, in real life it should have too.

But I'm kind of a weakling. And when I say kind of, I mean I have never picked up anything heavier than a tablet, and that my, uh, physique reflects that. I mean, can you blame me? My job is reading and research, and if I'm ever in the field it's supposed to be standing behind a burly tech mage in full spellarmor.

That's what they promised back at the academy, anyway.

I kicked as hard as I could manage, and the grate groaned. I kicked again and it bent slightly. Nine exhausting kicks later the grate clattered into the corridor beneath me.

I paused to catch my breath, then gently lowered myself through the opening, down to the deck. I might not be strong, but I am pretty damned agile. Just good enough to get frustrated when someone really good shows me up.

The rusted door glowed before me, the runes flickering unevenly under a thick layer of dark grime. The dialect was familiar, though the style was more archaic than what I was used to. I tapped the comm affixed to my collar. "Sapphire, I've got confirmation. This is definitely a storage locker, though I can't say for sure if it's an armory."

I sincerely hoped it was. Nothing was as valuable as weapons, not even lost knowledge, and every library on Kemet had a bounty on ancient books or knowledge scales.

"Can you get the door open or not?" Sapphire came back, not bothering to mask her impatience. I could hear the high-pitched whine of a laser torch behind her, and wondered what she was trying to open.

"Probably," I offered, though I wasn't in any way certain I could do what I was promising. "I'll get to work on it."

It went without saying that I wouldn't be able to carry whatever I found. I mean, I did have the infuse strength spell, so I could make myself stronger. But my strong was someone else's normal, and if there were rockets or other ordnance I wasn't going to be able to carry them alone.

The rest of the squad had each been given similar assignments throughout this level of the ship, the idea being that one of us would find something. Maybe more than one. Then we'd focus our efforts wherever the payoff was.

I bent to inspect the runes, which were straightforward enough. The lock was maintained by a separate spell, and the keypad basically counter spelled the lock when the correct combination was entered.

In theory, at least.

In practice, half the runes had faded to illegibility, which meant many of the input options were inoperable. If I was going to get inside, not only would I have to repair the panel, but I'd also have to somehow determine the locker's combination.

Normally that would be impossible, and we'd have to turn around and go home. Thank the lady for the magic I'd inherited from my mother.

I extended a finger, and concentrated. A thin sliver of *dream* crept up my arm, tingling as it reached the end of my finger. *Dream* magic is ephemeral, exactly as you'd expect.

Repairing the keypad required *air* magic, but *dream* would allow me to mimic *air*. As far as the console was concerned...it had exactly what it needed. Now I just needed to repair the missing runes.

That was going to be trickier. Most holodramas make it sound absurdly easy to pick a lock, but the truth is that you need a laser-torch and a whole lot of time to get into a vault like this. You can't just puzzle out a code by putting your ear against the wall.

Unless you happen to be an academy-trained flame reader.

I willed *fire* to move down my other arm, hot and urgent, and commanding release. I cupped my hand before my face, and a blue flame sprang up over my palm.

The flame undulated and danced, its rhythm a counterpoint to my heartbeat. I focused on this location, this place, which I was already familiar with, since I was literally standing in it.

Time became fluid. The clock ticked backward, in the flames at least. The image flickered wildly as years rolled backward into decades, and then a full century, but I didn't see any difference.

I jumped back a full thousand years, a significant length of time, in my opinion, and was mildly surprised to see most of the damage was still there.

A few of the runes were brighter, but several had already burnt out. This damage was older than I'd thought. Much older.

I pulled more *fire*, and a bit more *dream*, and willed my little flame to show me this same room ten millennia ago. The panel was bright now, though a few of the glyphs had begun to fade, heralding the damage I'd seen in the present.

A knot began to grow between my temples, the first throes of the migraine I'd earned for pushing my limits like this.

I took several deep breaths and allowed time to roll back slowly, a month at a time. It took three more jumps before I found what I was seeking.

A woman in a dark blue uniform with gold trim clutched

at her side as she hobbled up to the armory door. A deep pool of scarlet bled through her uniform over the gut, and her teeth were gritted in pain. She raised a trembling, bloody hand to the console and meticulously tapped a series of six sigils.

I watched them with rapt attention, memorizing each one as she pressed it, both the location on the pad and the appearance of the sigil. I'd need both to pull this off.

I rewound the timeline back to the beginning and watched it again, despite the cost in pain. Deep throbbing occupied the space behind my eyes, but it was worth it. I was positive I had it.

"Sapphire, this is Jerek," I mumbled into the comm. "I've got the sequence. I still need to repair the panel, but I might be able to get this thing open. Stand by."

"Really?" She sounded surprised. "Let me know how it plays out."

I bent to the panel, and extended a gloved hand, just as the woman had done all those millennia ago. Instead of touching the darkened sigil, I pulled at the reservoir of *dream* in my chest, just a sliver.

The magic lit the tip of my finger, and I sketched the sigils exactly as I'd remembered them. Traces of the earlier sigils remained to confirm my memory, and sigil by painstaking sigil I repaired time's ravages.

At last, an eternity and one backache later, I finished the last sigil. The panel lit up, and I couldn't help but grin.

I carefully typed in the sequence the woman had used, holding my breath as I did it. I had no idea how long had passed between the time the woman had opened the door, and the battle that had orphaned my ancestors. They could have changed the door code any number of times.

I was gambling they hadn't. People tend to follow the

path of least resistance, and that meant not changing an obscure armory code unless they absolutely had to.

K—thunk.

The door popped open with a hiss of stale air, exposing a room no one had seen since before my ancestors had made planetfall.

2

I leaned into the armory door, and was shocked by how heavy it was. Forcing it open enough to slip inside took almost thirty seconds of grunting and sweating. When I saw how thick the metal was, some sort of unfamiliar alloy, I understood why. A meter of dense metal could probably stop anything short of capital weapons or targeted explosives.

Inside the armory lay a modest room filled with some of the most valuable cargo in the sector. Two racks of spellrifles lined one wall, while a shelf full of fist-sized grenades ran underneath the rifles.

The opposite wall contained six suits of body armor constructed from an unfamiliar polymer. It resembled muscle, the texture at least, and was a deep charcoal in color. The suits lacked helmets, which seemed an odd oversight.

I moved to the armor first, and leaned closer to peer behind it. The armor wasn't bolted to the wall. It was held aloft through faint gravity magic, which had somehow survived all this time.

I wrapped both hands around the armor and pulled it loose, then nearly toppled under the weight. It was scout-class armor, and the material wasn't especially heavy, but I still struggled with it.

You might be asking yourself why it was worth the trouble if I'm such a wimp. Well, scavengers added a standard clause to all contracts centuries ago.

Anything you find that you can both use *and* carry belongs to you.

Find a pistol? Or a rifle? Or some armor? If you can use it, and carry it, then it's yours. The law was put into effect because mercs had effectively been forced into slavery, renting their own gear, and keeping nothing they found.

The back of the armor parted of its own accord, making it easy to pull over my flight suit. I did so, and wrestled awkwardly into the thing until all four limbs were where they were supposed to be. I felt like an idiot, and every step took a lot of effort.

I could deal with it. Long enough to get back to Kemet and sell it anyway. I looked around the armory, and tried to find anything else I might be able to carry. It would have to be small, or there was no way I'd be able to handle the hike back to the ship.

There was a rack of pistols under the rifles. I knelt next to it and inspected them. They were about the same size as Ariela, but where my pistol had a thicker bore with two muzzles, these were a bit slimmer with just one.

"Looks like it's designed solely with spells in mind," I muttered as I withdrew a spellpistol from the rack and belted it around the armor's thigh. I tucked my pistol into a belt on the other side, which made me look like a six-year-old's rendition of a gunslinger. A six-year-old on acid.

I considered taking some explosives too, but that was pushing it. The rest of this stuff would keep until I could make it back.

I leaned my chin down to activate the comm. "Sapphire, I've made it inside the vault."

"Don't enter until I get there," came back immediately.

"A little late for that." I couldn't help but laugh. "There's plenty for everyone. More than we can carry. Small arms and suits of body armor, all pristine."

"Nice work." The words were grudging, and I knew she'd be deeply annoyed when she saw what I'd taken. Sapphire wouldn't let go of a single credit, once she'd set her sights on it. And I was about to walk away with several thousand more than she'd expected. "I'll be there in ten. In the meantime—"

A high-pitched squealing came over the comm, and I winced as it tore through my temples. My last thought before I lost consciousness was that the timing couldn't be a coincidence.

I don't know how many seconds passed, but as I blinked away shards, I realized Sapphire should have said something by now. There was nothing. Was her comm damaged?

"Kid? Captain is gone. Lurkers." Wilson's gravelly voice came over the comm, soft as death. "If you can hear me get someplace dark and quiet. You're about to have incoming. At least four on the ground. Probably a lot more."

"Oh, crap," I growled, pacing through the armory as I tried to figure out what to do. Should I risk answering? I decided it was worth it, and pressed my chin against the comm to activate it. "I'm here, Wilson. I can lock myself in the armory. There's no way they'll get through that door."

"Sure, you could do that," his quiet voice came back.

"How much you got in the way of rations? Lock yourself in there, you're as good as dead. You know who this has to be."

"Lurkers, probably, like you said," I allowed. He was right. Staying in there probably was death. Besides, if I closed that door I might not be able to get it open again. "Change of plan. I'm going to leave the armory door open so they can get in."

"Don't do anything stupid, kid." Wilson's voice had somehow gone even more soft. "I'm gonna warm up the engines. You got until those bastards finish in that armory, and then I'm gone. Best get back quick. I told the others the same. I'm leaving the second they're done, or I see trouble, whichever comes first."

"I'll be there." I squeezed through the armory door and peered up the corridor. I couldn't hear anything yet, but they'd be here soon.

I trotted exactly three steps, discovered how heavy the armor was, then slowed it down to a walk. That meant lumbering up the hallway, knowing that enemies were approaching, and that if they heard a single clanking step I was done.

"Think, damn it." I stopped, and realized my heart was thundering and my legs were burning. I wasn't built for this kind of exertion. That was supposed to be the muscle's job, which we'd brought a lot of.

I had a little magic left, though my growing headache said I needed to be careful how I spent it, because I was going to need some serious downtime soon.

I channeled a little *fire* through my body, temporarily enhancing my strength. The spell wouldn't last long unless I fed it more magic, but it would last long enough to get me out of earshot.

My clanking steps came faster than before, and I hurried down one corridor, and up another. Finally I stopped and rested against the wall. A thick sheen of sweat coated my face and neck, and less pleasant areas. I really needed to start working out, assuming I lived.

"Okay," I reasoned aloud, keeping calm. "The lurkers are making for the armory. Once they find it they have no reason to look for me. I'm no threat. The *Remora* is though. They know we're here, and will attack the ship when it tries to leave."

I lurched into motion again, and started a winding path trying to work my way back to where we'd docked. I hadn't made it far when the math became inescapably clear.

No matter how fast I ran I wasn't going to make it back to the ship before the others. I closed my eyes, and relaxed as I activated the comm. At least I wouldn't have to run any more. "Wilson? I'm not going to make it."

"That sucks, kid." His gruff voice sounded a bit more tender than usual. "Anyone else got a line on us?"

"Wait for us!" came Erica's voice. "Davvyd and I are almost there. Need forty seconds."

"All right." Wilson perked up. He'd already written me off. "Get inside, and we'll get—"

I switched the comm off and closed my eyes. The full weight of what was happening hit me, and I sagged to my knees in the middle of the corridor.

They were leaving me behind. I was going to die.

My whole body seized up, and I fought back the tears. Everyone who'd told me I'd amount to nothing—had they been right all along?

Maybe. But if they were, I was still going to die on my feet, damn it. It was better than just lying there.

I climbed back to my feet and kept trudging up the corridor until I reached a T-intersection, then climbed a steep stairwell to the next level. That ended at a wide glass window that overlooked the hangar bay where we'd arrived.

I wasn't even sure why I was still going there, since I'd arrive too late. Maybe I just wanted to see them off.

"Thank the lady," I murmured, resting against the top of the stairwell as my heart rate returned to normal.

The *Remora* sat on the far side of the hangar, a good three hundred meters away. It may as well have been light years. As I stared in resignation her engines rumbled to life, and the corvette lifted off.

There was no waiting lurker vessel, or at least none that I could detect. They'd have docked somewhere in order to loot the armory, and that was the *Remora*'s one chance. If they could get away before the lurkers got back to their ship, then the lurkers probably wouldn't bother chasing them.

I held my breath as the *Remora* passed through the shimmering blue field that separated the docking bay from the frigid vacuum. They were going to make it.

They accelerated quickly, dipping under a torn girder, then out into open space. Even though they'd left me behind, I was happy they were getting out of there.

I was about to flip the comm back on to say goodbye when I spied movement in the black. Two rusty frigates, mismatched but no less lethal for it, emerged from cover to flank the *Remora*. They'd planned their ambush well.

Both vessels fired gauss cannons, which used magnets to hurl a hunk of metal at incredible speeds. Crude, but effective and inexpensive.

Two hunks of unprocessed ore slammed into the *Remora*'s main engine, which detonated spectacularly.

She went into an uncontrolled spin, but both lurker

vessels moved into a synchronous orbit and attached to her hull, one ship near the engines and the other the bridge.

I went cold. Every relic hunter knew that lurkers were thorough, and didn't leave crews behind. No one knew what they did with the bodies.

Maybe I'd gotten the better end of the deal after all.

3

I cannot express the horror that overwhelmed me in that moment. I stood there quivering, gazing helplessly at the pair of lurker vessels attached to the *Remora* like parasites. Wilson and Erica and Davvyd and Sapphire...gone. They hadn't been friends, but they'd been alive and now...just gone.

So how would I avoid the same fate?

I slumped over the railing, and tried to ignore the tears. It's not like anyone would see me breaking down, but I still felt embarrassed. I'd been trained, and now I needed to use that training. Not cry and piss myself like a child. My instructors back at the academy would be horrified.

So my first op had gone awry. I was still alive, and until that wasn't the case anymore I needed to deal with each problem as it appeared.

My breathing calmed, and the pain in my legs subsided to a dull ache. I considered my options. It didn't take long, because there weren't many. Either I needed to find an escape pod, a near impossibility on a vessel this close to the fringe, or I needed to hitch a ride on a lurker ship.

As I mulled those options over, my salvation strode into view. Two burly men in scored body armor struggled out of a corridor carrying a crate, which I guessed must contain the rifles and body armor I'd given them access to.

And if they were bringing it here...then they were expecting to get picked up. Of course they were. The *Remora* had been subdued. There was no danger. Why not use our LZ? In fact, why not bring our own ship back to haul the cargo, once they'd done for the crew?

My whole body went cold. Even as the thought flitted through my head I knew it was true. And, as expected, the *Remora* began slowly limping her way back into into the hangar bay, the hull shimmering through the blue field.

A plan began to form.

The lurkers would load the cargo, and then they'd board the ship, and then they'd leave...and head back to wherever they'd come from.

In the holos that would be some seedy base on the back of an asteroid somewhere, but in reality that wasn't feasible. No, they'd need a base with atmo and that meant they'd eventually be returning to Kemet.

I had to be on the ship when it left.

That was going to be more challenging than it sounded, unless I could come up with a clever workaround to being in terrible shape. I needed to cross a three-hundred-meter hangar in the time it took them to lift off.

Once I got there I needed to find a way into an airlock, and I needed to pray that it didn't trigger an alarm the lurkers were monitoring. What could possibly go wrong?

My first dilemma was the armor. The stubborn pragmatist in me argued that my chances were higher if I ditched it, but the miserly scavenger in me couldn't walk away from several thousand credits, especially given that I was in debt.

I still had some *fire* magic. I could juice my strength and run. My father had always argued that you could force your body to do things. That the secret was your mind. That if you learned to embrace pain, then you could push past anything.

Guess I was about to find out if he was right.

The pair of lurkers walked their crate up the ramp into the *Remora*'s cargo hold. I winced when I saw the dark stain on the metal. Someone had bought it in the cargo hold.

Another pair of heavily armored lurkers emerged from deeper in the derelict with another crate, and followed the first pair inside the *Remora*.

I counted under my breath, and fifty-four seconds later the first pair emerged. Seventeen seconds later the second pair emerged and headed back the way they'd come.

I'd used the air ducts to reach the armory, but they were going via the ship's corridors. That would take something like ten minutes, one way. I wasn't religious, but that had to be the maker watching out for me.

A turbo lift stood a dozen meters away, which would get me into the hangar. If I could cross the hangar in less than twenty minutes I could sneak inside the ship before they got back.

I lurched into motion and found a comfortable walking rhythm. It was hard, but manageable, even without the infuse strength spell. I grunted with each step, and thought about my father's disappointed face if I didn't make it home.

I doubted he'd mourn me for too long, but he would be disappointed that his son hadn't followed in his footsteps and made a name for himself. I loved my father, but he'd made it clear at an early age that my responsibility was to eclipse him.

The lift had a simple panel, and I pressed the down

arrow. It whirred into motion, and the platform floated down a level. I exited, and passed through a blue membrane into the cargo hold's dimly lit expanse.

"There's no way this is going to work," I muttered, as I forced myself into motion.

Twelve steps later I paused, and channeled my final infuse strength. I'd wanted to wait longer before using it, but my limbs were screaming and I didn't know how far willpower alone would take me.

The spell helped, and I settled into an easy trot that was anything but. Every step sent shards of agony further up my shins, and into my knees.

Adrenaline masked the pain, enough for me to soldier on, anyway. My father's growling voice echoed in my ears, and I trotted ever closer to the *Remora*.

My biggest fear, that a guard would emerge or one of the lurkers would return, was unfounded. I crossed the hangar, and reached the *Remora*'s blessedly cool hull.

"Oh, lady, no..." Horror bloomed when I saw the pair of guards standing at the top of the ramp inside the ship.

Neither one noticed me, and I ducked out of sight before they turned.

I hurried around to the underside of the ramp, and paused to catch my breath as my heart thundered in my chest. Exhaustion pulsed a counterpoint to the pain, and despair welled up underneath it all.

What the depths was I going to do?

I couldn't sneak up the ramp. I had a little *dream* magic left, but the closest I had to an invis spell was camouflage. I'd fade into my surroundings, but if I moved, the spell would break, and it could only fool one sense. That was no good.

Could I somehow get inside one of the crates? No, they

were already on the ship, and the ones they were bringing were being carried by very alert guards.

I could ambush the pair of guards, and I might even take them down, but then what? Four more were coming back, and I didn't know how many more were already inside the *Remora*.

I huddled under the steps, my mind spinning. No solution presented itself. Was I going to die? This close to survival?

Should I turn myself over? Maybe lurkers didn't kill prisoners. Yeah, right.

Eventually the lurkers with the crates returned, and I heard grunts as they muscled their way up the ramp above me. Their booted feet thudded directly over my head, and disappeared into the *Remora*'s cargo hold.

Then the ramp began to retract, and exposed my cowering form. Thankfully no one was there to see it. They were all safely aboard the ship that was about to carry them back to Kemet.

"No."

That one word sparked a deep resolve. I was going to live. I was going to find a way. I glanced down at my armor. There'd been no obvious helmet, but that seemed pretty stupid. It had to be better designed than that.

I closed my eyes and probed the armor with my magic. The armor gave a faint echoing answer, ready to receive whatever commands it had been enchanted with.

"I need a sealed environment, and internal life support." Issuing the order seemed like a child's nameday wish, and yet the armor responded. The wiry exterior slithered over my face, and a bright green HUD sprang to life.

I couldn't read the sigils, but the little blue cloud was

probably oxygen. That was good. Now I just needed a place to hold onto.

I looked up through the faceplate at the *Remora*'s landing strut, which would be retracting any second.

Now or never.

I stumbled over, and grabbed onto the strut. The ship began to rise from the deck, and the strut began to retract, with me attached.

"Please don't crush me!" I winced as the landing gear whirred shut, but I was folded into a comfortable area that might even have been air tight. It was too frigid for an unaugmented person to survive, but the armor might make it possible.

If, and only if, the lurkers were flying directly back to Kemet. If they really did have a secret asteroid base I had exactly as long as life support held out, and then I was dead.

4

The adrenaline began to fade as the ship rumbled into flight. I felt a momentary lurch, then things normalized as the *Remora*'s artificial gravity kicked in. Well, they normalized for an instant anyway.

"Errk." My face was suddenly pressed against the landing strut, and I couldn't lift it. The gravity was stronger this close to the hull, and well, we already talked about how strong I wasn't.

Thankfully, I still had the best defense an, uh, combat averse relic hunter can use. Sleep. I closed my eyes, and gave in to the inevitable. As darkness overtook me I idly wondered how long the life support would last.

I couldn't control whether I woke up or not. I'd done everything I could to make it this far. I'd earned a nap.

That nap went on for quite some time as it turned out. When I woke up, there was a puddle of drool under my right cheek and the HUD had changed. There was now an inflamed border to the whole thing, a pulsing angry red that made it very clear something critical was wrong.

I studied the HUD, and immediately spotted the problem. The little blue oxygen icon, a happy looking plant, was no longer happy. It had wilted into a near-lifeless brown shrub, and its roots were turning red. I don't know how that equated to time, but the message was clear. Life support was failing.

The air in the suit was a little stale, but only a little. I forced my breathing to slow, and relaxed a bit as my heart rate normalized. I had no idea how long I'd been asleep, but it had been long enough that my headache had faded to a dull throb. My legs burned, especially when I shifted in the armor.

"Okay," I muttered. I valued the oxygen, but sometimes talking to myself kept me moving. "How do I get out of this? I can't count on us arriving on any sort of timeline."

The problem loomed there, as another leaf fell off the dying plant icon. Shit.

"The life support is using magic. *Air* magic," I explained to myself, because self was in primitive-animal mode and needed a little TLC. "The ship let me repair a panel with *dream*. I have *dream*. Can I recharge the armor?"

I closed my eyes and probed my magic, which, as I mentioned before, lives in my chest. It's easiest to think of it like a hunk of radioactive matter that is now hardwired into my DNA. If I don't use my magic for a while that hunk will develop a skim of magic, sort of like radiation. That's how we power spells, but the closer mages run to dry the more it hurts.

I focused on that skim, the purple-pink mass I could feel, and fed a tendril of magic to the armor.

The HUD changed color immediately, and the angry red shifted to a rapidly flashing yellow. I kept up the flow of magic, and the flashing became less urgent, than stopped entirely.

I kept going, until the edge of the screen was once more tinged green. The oxygen icon had stabilized and now looked healthy once more.

I also noticed a change in another icon, though I had no idea what it did. The armor had a sort of paper doll icon, which I guess was meant to show me where battle damage happened. Above the paper doll was a golden crown that had been greyed out.

Now it was starting to turn yellow. Faintly still, but the icon had changed when I fed the suit magic. Interesting, but not nearly as interesting as the newly rejuvenated plant.

"Thank the lady," I muttered, eminently pleased with myself as I inhaled clean, fresh air. "Okay, now I can think out loud. So we're flying to their base, and we'll probably get there in something like eighteen to twenty hours given the *Remora*'s top speed, which they're probably using."

I had no way of knowing how long I'd been asleep, but I'd guess six hours? Something like that anyway. Theoretically I could sleep again, and when I woke up I could replenish the armor's oxygen one last time. That would keep me alive until they reached their base, but I'd have to be awake when that happened.

The seconds after the landing strut descended would be critical. I needed to get away from the ship and to a safe hiding spot before the ramp came down, or there was a good chance someone would see me.

There was also the chance that people might be waiting at the LZ, which meant I was boned no matter what I did. I had to ignore that possibility though, since I couldn't directly deal with it.

I channeled an infuse strength spell, and forced my armor into a more comfortable position. My whole body ached something awful. Not enough to keep me from sleeping though. I closed my eyes, and prayed that I was right in my estimates on our arrival.

Turns out I wasn't.

I slept right through the rest of the flight, and only woke up when the landing strut began to whir down. I blinked awake, realizing instantly that I'd somehow slept through re-entry.

Now or never.

I took a quick breath, then channeled an infuse strength spell. The armor became manageable, and the instant the landing strut crunched down on pocked concrete I started to run.

We'd landed on a weathered airstrip nestled in a small valley. A narrow road threaded up over the mountainside in the distance, and since that was the only way in or out of the compound I realized that would be where these guys would almost certainly be headed.

I ran the opposite direction, sprinting into the darkness toward the rocky hills in the distance for all I was worth.

Then the unthinkable happened. My foot caught on a cracked stone, and I careened forward. The armor insulated me from the pain of the fall, but I went skidding across the runaway in a shower of sparks.

Behind me the ramp was whirring into view. These guys were efficient, that was for depths damned sure. They were already clomping down the ramp in their mismatched body armor. That was interesting.

They hadn't claimed any of the cargo in the same way I had, which meant that whoever they reported to probably didn't honor mercenary salvage laws.

Strange thoughts given that I was on my ass out in the open, with hostiles approaching.

Thankfully, my extended nap had fully refilled my

magical reserves. I hadn't mastered advanced spells like invisibility, but I could use a simple camouflage spell. That had been the very first one most first-year boys learned back at the academy, and it had absolutely nothing to do with the girl's locker room.

I closed my eyes and channeled the spell. *Dream* swirled around me, and my armor took on the texture and appearance of cracked runway. I appeared to be an especially rough patch that most people would avoid.

Oddly, the little halo icon brightened again. Was it linked to me spending magic, even magic that didn't directly target the armor?

The *Remora*'s external lights began snapping on one by one, and for a single terrifying moment I wondered if they'd somehow seen me.

One of the flood lights splashed uncomfortably close, but being on the opposite side of the ship meant I was out of their direct field of view. If I lay there and didn't move, then I might be able to hide until they left. Then, theoretically at least, I'd be able to escape.

All I could do was wait. I lay there and watched as pairs of lurkers in mismatched environmental armor carried boxes onto a waiting transport, which was even more battered than they were. All their equipment was like that, ancient scavenged stuff that barely worked.

It looked like they'd either never gotten their hands on a decent haul, or more likely sold everything they recovered and lived frugally. I found it interesting that, from what I could see, anyway, lurkers were just scavengers who preyed on people instead of ships.

The holos made them out to be part monster, or maybe even another species altogether. They were larger than life and twice as scary. These guys? They were just bandits, really.

Then a pair of figures emerged wearing the same armor I had on, both with the helmets on so I couldn't make out faces. The leaders, apparently. They moved for the rover's pilot's compartment, separating them from the rest of the lurkers in the cargo hold.

I watched as they loaded the last of the cargo, and tried to ignore the knot between my shoulders. They were chatting amiably, though the *Remora*'s still cooling engines kept issuing metallic pings, which made it impossible to hear what they were saying.

The last of the lurkers loaded onto the transport, and the rover began the slow climb up the road and out of the valley.

I stared up at the *Remora*, and wondered if it really could be that simple. Had they not left any guards behind? I mean that might make sense, right? What would they need guards for? This place was remote, and the original crew was dead, at least as far as I knew.

I waited another fifteen minutes before moving, despite the mounting discomfort. My father had been right about that part at least. I could make my body do more than I'd thought, if my ass was truly on the line. Mind over matter and all that.

When I was absolutely certain the transport wasn't coming back I crawled to my feet and cautiously approached the *Remora*. The pinging of the engines had stopped, and the hum of the reactor had faded to a bare subsonic hum. That seemed like a good sign.

I crept around to the ramp, and peered up it. They'd left the running lights on in the hold, though the main lights were off. I'd be able to see, as would anyone still aboard...if anyone was.

The real question...was I brave enough to try taking back the ship?

My hand settled around Ariela, and I slowly withdrew the spellpistol from my holster. I had the second pistol as well, but unlike the holos I didn't think there'd be any advantage to using both at the same time.

I held the pistol before me with both hands firmly wrapped around the grip as my father had endlessly drilled me, and slowly advanced up the ramp. I tried to make each footstep as quiet as possible, and thankfully the wind outside helped mask the sound.

There were no alarming sounds from within. Nothing to suggest anyone was still aboard. My heart soared. If I was able to pull this off I couldn't even imagine my father's reaction.

Not only would I have survived, but I'd return home with cargo, and a ship of my own.

My fantasy died the instant I made it to the top of the ramp and saw the lurker standing at the far side of the hangar.

She was tall enough to look me in the eye, and wore thick, dark hair in a simple ponytail. The woman wore patched overalls with a homespun look to them, and from the grease stains I guessed maybe she was a mechanic. That didn't make her any less lethal.

The lurker had me dead to rights, with a well worn spellpistol trained on my chest. Apparently I hadn't been as quiet in my approach as I'd hoped.

I eased my finger onto Ariela's trigger, but that was a mistake. The lurker did what any smart merc would have done. She fired first.

A bolt of negative energy sizzled into my chest, slamming into the ancient armor. Much to my shock the armor absorbed the worst of the spell, and other than being knocked back a step and a light sunburn on my chest, I was unharmed.

I returned fire instinctively, and the spell I used reflected my training. A bolt of brilliant purple zipped from Ariela into the woman's face. It caught her squarely between her eyes, and the magic disappeared inside her skull with no visible effect.

At first anyway.

After a moment, her very pretty eyes fluttered shut, and she collapsed bonelessly to the deck.

I was about to cautiously advance when I heard a man's voice yell from deeper in the ship. "Hey, Vee, we need to get this thing locked up. We're going to be here for a while, at least until—"

The voice was getting closer, and I realized that I had no idea how many people were still on this ship. If this guy was the last one, maybe I could take him. Or maybe I'd die in the process. Maybe he had three more friends.

I turned on my heel, and fled back down the ramp. I had the armor and a sidearm. The ship was just gravy, and I'd rather have my life.

5

I sprinted down the ramp, and activated another infuse strength without slowing down. Under any other circumstances I'd have paused to congratulate myself, but I had a feeling I was about to have company.

The area around the base of the ramp was mostly clear, so I cut sharply to the left and used the ship as cover, exactly as my father had taught me. Always find hard cover, then set up a firing lane.

I knelt next to a landing strut, which provided partial cover. Ariela was still in my hand, but I gripped her with the other hand as well, and put her in a loose firing position. I'd still need to snap the pistol up, but if I sat in that position for too long my arm would cramp. Action hero I am not.

As expected, a set of boots clumped down the deck. A tall man with a thick auburn beard, not much older than me, spun around in a slow circle with a rifle cradled in his arms. An Inuran spellrifle from the look of it, though the barrel was scored and discolored.

Inuran tech was rare, as it originated in another system and only showed up when an Inuran trade moon happened through the Kemet system. That was rare enough that my father had to struggle to describe the last one, when he'd been four years old.

"Alpha, delta, get out here!" the lurker bellowed. "Someone took out Vee, and they're still close."

Instinct took over. I snapped the pistol up and sighted down the barrel. My target was standing still, and I wasn't a bad shot, so tagging him in the back with a dream bolt was easier than expected. The purple spell zipped into his back, rippling through his environmental armor and out of sight.

I didn't stick around to see if it took hold. It didn't matter. It was possible this guy was bluffing, and that there was no one else in the ship. It was possible my spell would take him out, and that I'd have won the day. But I had no way to verify any of that.

My father's gravelly voice offered clear instruction in my head. *Get clear if you aren't certain.*

So I got clear. I sprinted away from the ship, and ducked past the broken chain fence, into the scrub brush beyond. My infuse strength spell would last a while yet, and while it was active the armor was—

The golden halo brightened, and a flash came from the icon. Suddenly, a second, greyed-out icon appeared beneath the halo. Some sort of trident.

At the same time powerful magic rippled inward from the armor. It touched something inside of me, and left an... awareness in its wake. Some sort of link. I could *feel* the armor in a way I couldn't before.

Instead of a suit of dense metal it was almost alive. It became lighter, and easier to maneuver. It was as if the armor wanted to obey, to assist my movements rather than have me carry it.

All of a sudden running up the hill was a little less terri-

fying and a little more exhilarating. Sprinting became effort-
less, at least compared to what I'd been dealing with ever
since putting on the armor.

I paused briefly to glance back at the *Remora* and the
lurker compound, but I saw no new lights and no movement. My buddy had apparently retreated back in the ship,
or been dragged by someone else. Either way it confirmed
that I'd made the right decision in fleeing.

Scanning above me with the armor I spotted a clear trail
leading up to a pass between two low peaks. If I could get up
I'd be able to see for hundreds of clicks.

I guided the armor into an ungainly trot, and started
bounding up the ridge, toward the pass. It took an
exhausting twenty minutes to reach it, which was approxi-
mately twelve years faster than I could have hiked it on foot.
The armor didn't tell me the elevation, but I guessed we
were pretty high up.

A quick glance skyward confirmed a piece of my location. I spotted Set, the moon of anger, low on the western
horizon. The Vagrant Fleet glittered high above me, dominating much of the southern sky. It wasn't too different than
looking from my own backyard, which meant I couldn't be
more than a thousand clicks away from home.

I redoubled my pace, and eventually arrived at a low, flat
pass between two ancient mountains I didn't recognize. On
the other side lay salvation. Not just one city, but many. All
glittered below me in a sea of unbroken sprawl, all clustered
around the monorail lines flowing around the continent.

Those monorails had been my school, friend, and transport since I was old enough to wave my hand over the terminal. The lady had smiled on me. I was almost home.

I had plenty of time to consider the implications as I
started down the other side of the mountain. It would take

all night to reach the road below, and then until midday to reach the closest station, unless I found someone to give me a ride part of the way.

If not for the armor I'd probably have already lain down, but somehow it was keeping the exhaustion at bay. Mostly. I wobbled as I walked, and my eyes kept threatening to flutter shut.

"So," I muttered as I walked, mostly to keep myself moving. "I can confirm that lurkers live among us. They're relying on bad holos, and a couple decent ones, to convince us that they're monsters. Or aliens. Or maybe the remains of whatever enemy put the Vagrant Fleet out of commission in the first place."

I kept walking as I chewed on that. Lurkers were people. Just normal bandits, who happened to be a touch less friendly than your average merc. My whole worldview had been upended, and as I approached the sea of glittering lights below I wondered how many of those people were lurkers. How common was this sort of thing?

It couldn't be profitable to stake out a random derelict at the edge of the fleet. That wouldn't make any sense. What if potential victims never showed? You'd spend a bunch of precious O_2, rations, and fuel, and for what? No, it only made sense if...if you were *absolutely certain* prey was about to arrive.

And the only way to be certain would be to know in advance that a flight plan had been filed with the ministry. Someone in the ministry was probably selling that information. Hell, if this was a holo, then maybe the minister herself was a lurker. Dun dun DUN.

The night passed slowly, and I spun out dozens of interesting conspiracy theories. That wasn't the only thing to occupy my interest though.

The armor itself was of great interest. I badly wanted to know what would activate the trident icon, and what that might do. Hopefully it was some sort of badass weapon. Or a pile of credits.

And was there another icon past that one?

Some of the more powerful mages walked around with staves that were apparently not only ancient, but also sentient magic items. Just like Ariela, but more advanced.

Ariela was capped, meaning she had no more room to grow. She was as cool as she was ever going to get.

But what about the armor? How cool was it going to get? What else could it do? On and on my mind went, but without some sort of user's manual or access to academy resources I couldn't learn any more about it.

By the time I reached the road, I was pretty much done with walking. Even though the suit had grown lighter, and the act was easier, it was just so damned boring. People ran for fun? By the maker, *why*?

I trotted up the road, each step sending up a puff of dust as I approached the towering monorail in the distance. I could see the tiny specks picking their way up the wide concrete stairs, toward the hundreds of landing areas that would whisk them across the continent.

No one looked twice at me as I joined the trickle of foot traffic. Transports screamed by overhead as they landed near monolithic parking structures, and if not for my helmet the noise would have been deafening.

I'd always hated crowds, but the armor provided a literal barrier, and I felt...well, more protected I guess. I walked with more confidence than I'd mustered just a few days ago.

People got out of my way as I mounted the stairs, which surprised me until I realized that the armor still had fresh battle damage. People could see I'd been shot in the chest with a void bolt, and that I was still moving.

Holy crap. These people were afraid of me.

I began a quite unmanly giggle, and hurried up the stairs, toward the automated kiosk. I had a chip implanted in my palm just like everyone else, and swiped it under the scanner as I entered the turnstile.

It would deduct over half my remaining credits, but the fare would carry me home, no matter how far out I was. I stepped through the turnstile, and hurried to the third floor, where my gate stood. As I walked over I glanced at the ticket that had been printed.

"New Cairo?" I muttered, a bit surprised. I'd heard of the sprawling southern capital, but had never visited. I glanced around, but couldn't catch sight of any of the pyramids that made this place famous.

For just an instant I longed for time to explore, but I needed to get home, and quick. I'd taken out a bond to cover my mission expenses, and I needed to pay it back by tomorrow, or it would go up by 20%. Every day.

I waited patiently, and an aging white hovertrain rumbled up. I slipped inside with a crowd of passengers, most of whom kept their distance. I guess with the dirt on the armor from my fall, and the dual pistols, and the battle damage, I must actually look like the real deal.

I decided to enjoy it, and casually rested my hand on Ariela's grip. The people around me tensed. I released the grip and folded my arms.

Yup, I'm kind of a bad ass...until I run into a real one.

INTERLUDE I

Matron Jolene strode into the minister's office with all the grace and dignity she'd earned over a lifetime of dealing with rulers and tyrants, from a position of strength.

She represented the Inuran Consortium, the sector's leading arms supplier, and one of its largest enigmas. They worked tirelessly and ruthlessly to keep anyone from knowing their fleet strengths, or even the location of their shipyards, much less their many magitech R&D facilities.

That was their way. Everything was cloaked in tradition and secrecy, an alluring combination to most outside cultures.

A pair of guards, both in tasteful suits with no obvious weaponry, flanked the minister's desk. Both eyed Jolene in open lust, one a man, the other a woman. That was unsurprising, and another advantage in the Inuran arsenal.

Unlike humanity, all Inurans were beautiful. They stood closer to the divine than lesser races, and those lessers sensed their place. That made dealing with them easier.

"Welcome, Matron." Minister Ramachan rose from

behind the desk, and offered a warm smile that highlighted her relative youth, forty-three, a tender enough age that even some humans had noted it during her campaign for the position. She had rosy skin of a darker hue that Jolene rather liked, as much red as brown. "Please, make yourself comfortable."

The minister gestured at a pair of plush chairs opposite her desk, and Jolene adjusted her business skirt as she moved to sit. She waved a hand, and her attendants flanked the doorway leading back the way they'd come.

That gave the appearance that this was a one-on-one conversation, between equals, although both parties knew that wasn't the case.

"Thank you, Minister." Jolene gave her a cool, judgmental smile. The effect was not lost. The minister's smile slipped a hair. "I appreciate your offer of accommodations, but I will be remaining on my flagship. I have traveled a long way, and am weary. Please, why have you sent for me?"

Jolene already knew the answer, of course. It had been her idea, after all. Orchestrated over the last five years all in preparation for this precise moment. A careful, quiet campaign of seemingly random chaos and misfortune, all driving the minister and her government in the direction Jolene wished.

"Call me Divya, please." The minister returned to her seat, and rested her hands on the mahogany desk, which lent her at least a little authority. "Matron, I will be frank. It's been over forty years since the last Inuran trade moon visited our system. We're using outdated, badly repaired tech. We lack enough *void* mages, as you know, so we can't use the Umbral Depths to travel."

"Which means a roughly two-year trip to the closest habitable system, yes?" Jolene folded her hands in her lap.

As always, she already knew the answer. She glanced out the minister's office windows, which afforded a magnificent view of the famed Kemet sunset. Pity all this would be gone soon.

"Four years," the minister continued, fixing Jolene with an intense gaze, one filled with intelligence, "will buy us a round trip to Sanctuary, a station at the edge of your sector. When we get there, we're overcharged for basic supplies, and can't bring back even a third of what we need, much less the luxuries our more wealthy mercenaries crave. The only time my best people get out of the system is when they join a long campaign in one of the sector's wars, but then they come home rich with nothing to spend their credits on."

Jolene gave her best approximation of a sympathetic nod, a fairly good one in her estimation. "I can see how a trade moon would benefit your people, but you must understand the difficult position this puts me in. The last time we visited the Kemet system we took in less than sixty percent of projected revenue. We barely paid for the trip, Divya. If I oversee a blunder like that again my board will remove me from power."

Her board was comprised of puppets and sycophants, of course. But the minister didn't know that. No one outside of the innermost Inuran ranks did, so she could make up whatever she wanted.

"I understand your reservations." The minister leaned back in a chair that absolutely dwarfed her, and that Jolene guessed had probably been chosen by her predecessor, as had the desk. Her dark hair framed dark skin, and the chair's leather backing enhanced the look. Quite charming, really. "I can assure you the trip will be profitable. We have two generations of wealth to spend."

"I believe you, Minister, but I cannot act without guarantees." Jolene put her hands up as if absolving herself of responsibility, as if she were not the absolute authority among the Consortium. "We all answer to someone."

"Of course, I understand the position this puts you in," Ramachan said, not a hint of reproach in her voice. "What sort of collateral can we offer to secure a visit in the next six months? Surely there must be something that would allay the fears of your board."

Jolene tapped her lip with a finger as if considering. "It would have to be of considerable worth. Moving a trade moon is neither quick nor economical."

"The collective service of the finest mercenary legions in the galaxy aren't enough?" Ramachan's eyes narrowed, and Jolene gained a small measure of respect for her. The minister knew the worth of her people, and it was considerable.

Thankfully, Jolene already had a way to steal Kemet's best and brightest for a fraction of their worth.

"We'd need more tangible collateral, I'm afraid." Jolene shook her head sadly. "My people only value hard assets. I cannot sell a deal based on future labor."

Ramachan nodded gravely, then leaned back in her chair, as if pressed back by the weight of her troubles. She seemed to consider something at length, and when the deliberation ended she looked up to meet Jolene's stare kilo for kilo. "What if I could offer the academy armory? We have over a dozen artifacts from the godswar. Weapons of tremendous age, worth, and power. The magitech is unrivaled."

Jolene didn't soften her patronizing smile. She probably should have, but the very idea of some backwater world

offering their trinkets up to the finest artificers the sector
had ever known... it was preposterous.

"Ahh, I'm sure your collection is impressive," Jolene
finally said. She couldn't force more respect into her tone,
but at least she could make the words palatable. "Unfortunately what you view as unrivaled technology we see as cast
off refuse from a time when the Consortium was still
learning how to perfect spelldrives. The devices in your
Highspire armory are valuable, from a historical perspective, but not to my people. We care little for history or your
people's legacy. You'd need to sell those items to a world like
Shaya, which is both wealthy and sentimental."

The minister sagged in her chair, defeated. She licked
her lips, and shook her head as if silencing some internal
thought. Jolene stilled a smile. As much as she enjoyed the
moment when an opponent broke she was also wary of
premature celebration.

She allowed the minister to twist for several moments
before she intervened.

Jolene leaned casually back in her chair, then blinked in
her carefully planned "aha" moment. "I have it! The Vagrant
Fleet. The mineral wealth alone must be fantastic, not to
mention the archeological value. If you're willing to offer
salvage rights to the Vagrant Fleet up as collateral...well, that I
can sell to the board. We won't ever need to collect on that, of
course. Provided you meet or exceed our modest sales goals."

The minister cocked her head and adopted a shrewd
look. She was smarter than Jolene liked, but in the end she
only had one viable option. The Inurans had carefully
starved the Kemet system, as they'd done to many systems
in the past.

That made a populace, and its ruler, desperate. And

pliable. Especially when they didn't see the hook. The minister clearly feared that Jolene was using this as a way to steal the only real asset outside of their precious armory that remained to these people.

"Come now, Minister," Jolene prompted, striking at the moment of indecision. "The fleet is thick with lurkers and pirates, more so every cycle. It isn't a viable source of revenue for your people and hasn't been for decades. In the unlikely event that you can't make the sales numbers, what do you really lose? Some ancient space hulks long picked clean?"

The minister was silent for a long time. Long enough that Jolene almost spoke again, though she sensed it would be a mistake.

"Very well," the minister finally agreed, though she looked as if she'd eaten something sour. "I can arrange to have a confederate bond placed against the fleet. In the event that we are unable to meet the sales target we will forfeit all salvage rights. As long as you give me a number I can hit, this can work out well for both of us."

"Of course," Jolene quickly agreed, offering her first genuine smile. "Let me assure you right now, minister, that those goals will be very achievable. The Inurans thrive on continued trade. Abusing our trade partners harms our reputation, and we'd never do that for some ancient derelict ships."

She would, however, do it to secure some of the most advanced technology the sector had ever seen. Jolene had lost much recently. Power. Prestige. Her place among the sector's wealthy and elite.

Her own daughter had become a goddess, and Voria would no doubt kill her on sight given that Jolene had sided with Skare and Talifax. So Jolene needed to make sure she stayed away from the blasted Confederacy.

Far away.

But she wasn't going to slink off into the shadows. She was going to retrofit a new fleet, one stolen from these yokels. Then, she'd take their finest troops and use them to carve out a new power base in a distant sector.

The cost was small. A single planet no one cared about.

6

The instant the train's doors hissed shut behind me I began to tremble. I didn't know why, but as I held a hand up for inspection I confirmed that it was shaking violently. I clenched it into a fist, and that seemed to still the episode.

For a moment.

It came back in full force, but now both my hands were shaking. An unfamiliar tension gripped my chest and my shoulders, tightening me into an ever smaller ball.

A quick glance around the train confirmed I was the only occupant in this car, which made sense given the hour. That was all the permission my body needed to break down.

Deep, wracking sobs rolled through my chest, and I began to ugly cry into the helmet. As the train sped along, familiar lights flashing above every hundred meters, I felt safe for the first time since I'd left Kemet.

I didn't know if it was decompression or some sort of post-traumatic stress, but I couldn't stop crying for a good three minutes. Eventually the sobs worked themselves out, and I was left trembling and sucking in deep lungfuls of air.

It made sense that there'd be an emotional toll, I suppose. I'd just never had to pay it before, and truth be told I wasn't handling it well. People I'd known were dead now, and if not for several incredible coincidences I would be dead too. My survival was nothing more than chance.

I shook my head, and tried to focus on other things. I didn't want to be in my head any more. I didn't want to think about what I'd gone through. So I focused on the terrain rolling by outside the train's darkened windows.

Wait, what was that?

I grabbed the support bar over my shoulder, and leaned a bit closer to the train's slanted windows. All along the western horizon the night was devouring the sky. On one side the sun was giving up its daily struggle, but on the other I could already see stars and the glittering edges of the Vagrant Fleet.

"What the—?" I leaned up against the glass as an object appeared on the horizon.

I still had my helmet on, and to my mild surprise the HUD put a reticle around the object, and a tag appeared with various forms of data. My ancient draconic was rusty, but I thought I was looking at the word "comet". One that seemed to be passing uncomfortably close to our world.

A small black halo appeared around the comet, and an angry beeping came from my armor. Red text began scrolling underneath the comet, fast enough that I felt compelled to cheat.

"Universas Solarus," I whispered, and the text instantly rearranged itself into much more familiar galactic standard.

Anyone staring at the same text would still see draconic, but the magic translated it into a form my brain could understand. All academy mages were bonded upon graduation, and could access any language known by even a single member. And collectively we knew pretty much all of them.

"Oh, crap," I muttered as I scanned the contents.

The black halo indicated *void* magic, apparently. That meant someone had been playing with gravity, someone powerful enough to mess with a rock the size of a small moon. At least, if my armor was right.

It could be some sort of malfunction. Maybe the rock just had some lingering *void* magic? The idea that someone or something could change the orbit of a celestial body with magic seemed...well, crazy.

Magic could let you blow a ship up. Or teleport. Or do all sorts of crazy things. But hurl a whole moon at a planet? I couldn't get my brain around it.

The text on my HUD seemed pretty clear, though, and if it was right, the final paragraph scared the depths out of me. I read it aloud: "Planetary orbit will decay until this world passes the Roche point. Violent geologic instability will precede planetary destruction."

Yeah, that seemed pretty grim. Suddenly my problems were beyond petty. At the same time my next step wasn't clear. What did I do with this information?

My hands began shaking again. Maybe they had never stopped, and were getting worse. I wrapped them around the support bar and squeezed to still the tremors.

No one in any position of authority knew who I was, and if I could detect this stuff, then the ministry had people that could do the same thing, right? I should stay out of it. If there were a real threat, social media would already be going orbital.

They didn't need some random brand new relic hunter still paying off academy loans to tell them how to run their world. But...if I was right, this impacted me too. And everyone I cared about.

The train slowed, then stopped. I exited onto the familiar 16B platform, then trotted down the grime-darkened stairs, into an alley that reeked of people refusing to die.

Layer after layer of freeways blocked out the sky above me, and only the occasional surviving streetlight kept the darkness from winning entirely. The shadows were deep and dangerous. All manner of thugs lurked there, but for the first time I didn't scurry back to my apartment.

I walked. No, I ambled. I took my time, and made it clear that I didn't care who knew where I was going. I understood the effect that would have, of course. Body armor wasn't uncommon, and seeing a suit you didn't recognize was mildly interesting, but not cause for alarm.

People would remember my passage, but hopefully they assumed I was too much trouble to bother with. That was the game we always played here. Either you avoided the gangs or you put up a brief front long enough to skirt their territory.

Either through luck or my bluff no one bothered me as I threaded down an alley, up the neighboring street, which was too choked with refuse for vehicles to pass, and then down another alley.

Every time I saw another landmark I breathed a little easier, and when I reached the flopstack where my father and I lived, the tension I'd been holding since I left home finally eased. I trotted up the rusted metal stairs, then waved my hand in front of the keypad outside our door.

The seal hissed open, and I ducked quickly through the rusted doorway. I glanced around behind me, and saw several curious neighbors watching. They'd talk, but there was little harm in what they could say. I closed the door, and leaned against the wall.

The creak of leather came from the next room. My dad in his recliner. "Jer, that you? Only been a week. That outfit o' clowns you signed up with void their contract that quick?"

Might as well get this over with. I took a deep breath, and willed the suit's helmet to retract. It slithered off my face, which was a little disorienting, but over quickly, thankfully.

I stepped into our living room, which was a three-meter cube constructed from super-dense plastic. Some families could afford five or six of the modular rooms, but dad had never been able to afford more than two. He lived in this one, and stored his junk in the extra one, where I happened to have a bunk.

Now, before you make any assumptions, my dad is a good guy. He just likes junk, and there's no crime in that. And, he'd always made sure I hadn't starved, which gave him high marks in my book, despite any personal beefs I might have. Part of why I wanted to succeed at this relic hunter thing was so that I could look after him instead of the other way around.

"Hey, Dad." I stood up straight, and moved to stand before the recliner that had become both home and prison after he'd lost both legs on his last op. "Made it back in one piece, and with some salvage."

Dad stroked his greying beard, a stark contrast to his bald pate, and sized me up with bleary eyes. He took a swig of his nanite-infused beer, a clever invention that repaired the kidneys and prevented hangovers. Wildly popular, as you might imagine.

"Don't recognize the make, and I've seen 'em all," my dad finally said. He scooted up a bit in his chair. "The pistol seems like standard issue. Might get you a couple hundred credits. You take out a bond?"

"Yeah," I admitted, shoulders slumping.

"How much?"

"Three thousand," I allowed. I knew how he'd react, but I'd learned long ago it was best to tell the complete truth and then wait out the storm.

"Why did you even go?" Dad finally choked out, eyeing me with those hateful eyes, the demon that always lurked underneath. "You got depths damned lucky that you found that armor, and that it might sell for a few thousand credits. You better pray it does, though why some moron would buy armor without a helmet I'll never know. I can't bail you out this time, and don't even think about calling your mother. She's got important academy stuff to be about, and doesn't need us inconveniencing her in her new life."

There it was. The root of the anger. This didn't have anything at all to do with me. It never had.

"You're right." I raised my palms in a placating gesture. "I got lucky. It wasn't my brightest move, but I'm still hoping I came out of it ahead a few credits." I paused, and considered what the armor had told me about the comet earlier. I was tired, but planetary destruction sounded pretty bad. "Was there anything on the news about that comet?"

"Yeah." Dad waved dismissively, and turned his attention back to the holo that dominated the far side of the cube. "Something about aftershocks, but that it will be gone in a day or two. I felt one of 'em here, but it wasn't bad. Not even sure why they felt the need to report it."

"I'm pretty beat from re-entry." I tried to keep my voice light, but was positive he picked up the quaver. My hands were shaking. Had the armor's warning been right? If it was, how long did we have? "I think I'm going to knock off early."

My father heaved a deep, and very familiar, sigh. He turned his "I'm disappointed again" face on, and speared me with his most judgmental gaze. "Son, you look like you're about to fall over. If you put in a few months at the gym it would change your life. You wouldn't be so tired all the time. I know you ignore most of my advice, and that you take after your mom with that giant brain. But that doesn't mean you have to be a weakling. Give it a chance, son, please. The iron will change your life."

"I will, Dad." I nodded, and slipped past him into the second cube, between the towering rows of junk. Doing so required me to squeeze past the weight set my dad still used religiously. I'd lost track of the number of jokes about skipping leg day since my dad, well, didn't have legs.

My father had been after me to go to the gym for over a decade, but I'd had some bad experiences, and hated that place. Working out alone seemed more my speed, but I'd always been afraid to try. What if I couldn't lift the bar and had to ask my dad for help?

I squeezed onto my bunk, and considered taking off the armor, but I really was exhausted. I drew my worn blanket over the armor, and laid my head on a pillow flatter than my bank account.

Home sweet home. Tomorrow, if the world was still here, then I'd deal with whatever "planetary destruction" meant.

Tonight I was out of gas, and sleep came quickly.

7

The next morning I woke up scratching myself. Everywhere. My whole body itched, and I thrashed desperately on my bed, unable to reach the source because I'd gone to bed wearing the armor.

Mind over body.

I forced myself to stop thrashing, and then to lay back against the bunk. *Breathe*. The itching continued, but I was getting better at resisting it.

"Okay," I muttered. "Time to get some answers."

I willed the helmet to cover my face, and it did. Thankfully the itching didn't spread, and seemed confined to below the neck. After a moment the HUD lit, and I inspected the readout.

The paper doll hadn't changed, but a little wheel had appeared next to the crown and trident. It was spinning, and looked different than the other icons. A progress indicator.

The color changed with each pulse, beginning a deep, angry red, and slowly lightening to green. The itching never let up, but having something to focus on made it a whole lot easier to keep calm.

What was the armor doing to me? That had to be it. No other explanation made sense. Unfortunately, I still lacked a manual and couldn't really ask the armor. That meant I just had to wait it out, then try to understand what it was doing to me. Hopefully it wasn't irradiating my junk.

The spinner finally turned a bright, happy green, then winked out of existence. The itching vanished instantly. My breathing eased, but my whole body trembled. I wasn't sure I could stand up if I needed to, and I didn't even know why.

"Dad," I called weakly, my throat raw and voice hoarse. There was no answer. I closed my eyes and slowly counted to twenty, then opened them again.

Did I feel any different? A little. My limbs felt like they had after our physical endurance training back at the academy. I'd hated running, and how it made my whole body ache afterwards. That was how I felt, times about a million. Literally every part of my body hurt.

Well, not literally, but certainly enough to make me abuse the word.

I sat up with a groan. It took effort, but it didn't hurt. Why did everything ache so badly?

"Armor," I begged, knowing it was futile. "What did you do to me, and why?"

Text began scrawling across the bottom of the screen, in draconic of course. *Celeritas Invegra*. Some sort of accelerated bio-enhancement spell? I pushed a stack of boxes out of the way, which was easier than it should have been.

That exposed a mirror I seldom had cause to use, but under a layer of dust I could see myself. See the changes. The armor was the same, but the corded suit was form-fitting, and the form it fit had changed.

I had muscles. Not big ones, mind you, but visible

muscles. I'd gone to bed with arms like tube sausages, flat and shapeless, and woken up with a recognizable triceps.

That was way, way too good to be true. If I exited the armor what would that do to me? The magic, whatever it was, had to be temporary. There was no way to permanently alter the human body like that, or if there was it was stronger magic than I'd run across. I hadn't seen everything, after all. And the academy didn't know everything.

Fortunately, I had a far more terrifying problem to deal with. I needed to figure out whether or not our world was actually in danger, and if so, figure out who I could tell that would make even the slightest bit of difference.

At the same time, I had the more immediate problem of needing to pay off my bond. Trying to save the world with debt-collecting hit men after me did not seem smart. I had until the end of business, and if I didn't have the credits by then, well...it wouldn't really much matter to me if the world blew up.

I turned back to my bed and fetched my backpack from underneath, then slung it over one of the armor's shoulders. I unzipped it, and noted the water bottle was still half full. That should be enough for today, if I avoided the sun and didn't exert myself too heavily.

I could buy more, but my account was already in the red zone, and I'd just as soon sell the armor and see where I stood. I headed back into my father's flop, and gave him a bro-nod.

He had no choice but to return it, and said nothing to me as I crept past him and through the flop's already open door. My father knew what I had to do, and while he didn't offer encouragement, at least he hadn't told me I couldn't do it, as he sometimes did. To my mind that meant he was rooting for me.

I paused outside the door, testing the air with both nostrils. Just the usual rank sludge, thank the maker. I'd learned early on what blood smelled like, and if it was around, I didn't want to be.

Once outside the flop, I willed the helmet to slither over my face, then cautiously left the alley for the cracked thoroughfare. There weren't very many places I could go, which made the choice easy.

I needed a friendly face, one I could unload on, who would not only not mind but would appreciate being involved in something interesting.

That meant Briff, my best friend from the academy. We'd come up together through the ranks, and had formed an arena team that had dominated our senior year. Now we both fervently hoped that hadn't been the peak of our careers that we fondly reminisced about when we were old and even more destitute.

The op on the *Remora* had been my first job after graduation. So far as I knew, Briff hadn't gotten a job. He'd somehow remained in his academy dorm, and was living there rent free until they figured it out.

I hoofed it up the boulevard, and turned north. The walk to the academy was about eight clicks, which would take most of my morning. And give me too much time alone in my head thinking about things I'd just as soon avoid admitting I knew.

I waved my hand, and an automated lift zoomed over. I slipped into the tiny vehicle's sole compartment, and hadn't even buckled my harness before it shot back into traffic.

"Input destination, please," a pleasant feminine voice came from the vehicle's dashboard.

"Take me to the academy. Drop me off as soon as you hit the campus." I'd added that last order because if I didn't the lift would find the exact center of the campus, and roam around while racking up charges I couldn't afford.

I relaxed into the hard plastic seat as much as I was able to, but each time we darted through traffic and passed another lift my mind flashed back to the dreadnought. To hiding in the strut. To seeing those ships come for the *Remora*.

Thankfully we reached the campus within a few minutes, and the lift deposited me on the sidewalk. I followed it to block four, which was the closest building, a four-story dormitory designed to hold about a thousand students.

I waited for a distracted young woman to leave, then darted over to the door before it closed. I seized it just in time, and slipped inside the dorm. We'd perfected the practice during our freshmen year, as we often came home after curfew and didn't want a record in the system.

The stairwell was next to the door, so I ducked inside and followed it up to the fourth floor. I poked my head out of the stairwell, but there was no sign of campus security.

Briff's door was the second one on the left, and had been mine for about two years as well. I missed the place, and was shocked to see how little furniture remained in the tiny two-bedroom apartment. The place was...empty.

A familiar two-meter plus dragon lounged on what remained of a couch that had clearly been designed for humans. His left thumb and forefinger tapped furiously at the air; the motion picked up the console and instantly translated into his character firing on the holographic projection over the device.

"Hey, Briff," I called from the doorway, waiting for acknowledgement. "Is it cool if I come in?"

"Oh yeah, man," Briff's slitted, draconic irises never left

the holoscreen and I slipped inside the flop. It was notice-ably warmer. Unpleasantly so.

Briff's character took a void bolt from behind, and went down, and the screen flashed defeat and then a scoreboard showing Briff's performance...which wasn't half bad.

"You've been improving." I pulled up an empty vat of algae and flipped it over as a seat. My only option other than the floor, since I saw no furniture outside the holo and the couch.

"Been playing a lot since graduation." Briff delivered a toothy grin, exposing rows of deadly teeth. The threatening image was ruined by the rather substantial gut he'd managed to accumulate, and the pile of discarded energy drink cans littering the floor around his couch. "Maybe a little too much. Got myself a really good team, and we were just wrecking arena. Felt like you and I back at the academy. I'm telling you...we'd have gone pro if we'd kept after it."

"Maybe," I allowed, and meant it. We'd had the right mix of intelligence and instinct, and among the five of us, had dominated the academy's tourney that year. "But we didn't keep after it. And only you and I are left. Mala left during the last hiring, and Roktar the one before that."

"Well," Briff rumbled as he waved his scaly hand and the holo went into standby, "at least I've been able to pretend for the last couple days. Sooner or later they're going to kick me out. Sooner, I think. A campus goon came by earlier to disconnect quantum, but I faked a molting and he left. So how did your trip go? Did...depths, man, what are you wear-ing? Did you guys strike it big? Tell me everything!"

Briff's leathery wings gave a short flap as he lumbered up onto two legs, and took a step closer to me. The dormitory's floor groaned in protest, and I imagined the students below were terrified whenever Briff came or went.

The hatchling leaned closer, and tilted his head to inspect the armor. "Wow. Oh, wow. This isn't recorded in the codex. This is new. If you auction this, and invite some professors from the armory...depths, maybe have your mother pull some strings and get the minister to attend. This belongs in some fancy museum or maybe the armory itself, and you need to line your pocket."

Only the most amazing, ancient, and unique artifacts were placed in the armory, our planet's repository of magitech, mostly passed down from the battle preceding planetfall.

That answered my first question. No one knew weapons and armor like Briff. No one. That he was impressed backed up my own findings, but also made the weapon's ominous prediction more likely to be true.

As if summoned by the thought, the entire building began to shake violently. I tumbled into the wall, then landed in a pile of empty cans as the entire building swayed backed and forth. The earthquake went on for a good thirty seconds, then ceased abruptly.

"That was even worse than yesterday," Briff groused as he pulled himself to his feet. Apparently the dormitory floor was stronger than it looked, if it had survived that. "Every time it happens it knocks out quantum. Now I gotta wait before I can get online again. You'd think the academy would have a better connection." He heaved a heavy sigh, then dropped down onto the couch, which strained, but held.

"Briff, you said you wanted to hear how I got the armor?" I began, knowing that was the way to secure his interest. "I found it on a derelict dreadnought. One of the Great Ships. It was inside a weapons locker that hadn't been opened since before planetfall. A long time before planetfall."

Briff's eyes widened, and his tongue played over his teeth in a way that had always unnerved me. Like a dragon surveying something it was about to eat. At least he was interested.

"And?" Briff demanded.

"And it came from the height of the dragonflight epoch, maybe seventy thousand years ago." I willed the helmet to slither over my face, and it obliged. "Look at me, Briff."

I extended my arm, and made a motion that terrified flaccid guys like me everywhere. The one designed to show off your biceps. I flexed. This time...I actually had a muscle.

"Depths, man. Is that built into the armor? You look like you've been working out all summer." Briff's tail began swishing back and forth, knocking the holo off its stand, which even the earthquake hadn't managed to do. The plastic device cluttered to the carpet, forgotten for the moment at least. "Tell me, man. I have to know."

"The armor magically induced my muscles to grow," I explained. I didn't understand it well, but I still tried to boil it down quickly. "It's advanced in ways I didn't realize were possible for magitech. You can see what it did to my body in just a couple days, right? You're with me on that?"

"Okay, so it's advanced. And it should be in the armory." Briff finally took a step backwards, reining in his interest. "You're getting to a point, and I have a feeling I'm not going to like it."

"Briff, those quakes?" I stabbed a finger out the dormitory's door, at the world at large. "They're going to pull this planet apart. The armor is convinced of it. That comet destabilized our orbit. Bad things are going to happen."

"Huh." Briff calmly returned to his couch, his wings flapping furiously as he settled his bulk. "Well, that sucks."

"That's it?" I protested. "You're just going to sit there and play virtual arena? I just told you the world is ending."

It was the first time I'd said it out loud, and it sounded just as crazy as I feared it would.

The way Briff was looking at me didn't suggest disbelief. It was resignation. He shook his scaly head, sadly. "If you're right, let's say we've got a week. What am I going to do? I can sit here and play arena, feasting on algae, or maybe even some soy steaks. Or, I can panic and run around frantically, and then still die. In a way this is good news. Now I can blow off my shift tonight. Do you have any idea how boring being a security guard is?"

"You don't even want to know how the world is going to end?" My shoulders slumped. I thought I had an ally.

"Nope." Briff's tail curled around the holo, and set it back on the stand. "You can hang out if you want, but I'm not leaving unless that campus goon comes back."

Guess I needed to solve this on my own.

8

I left Briff's dormitory with my head spinning, but not so much so that I abandoned caution. I caught a lift back to the flopstacks, knowing that would make me a target as I exited. A whole industry has formed around hitting returning drunks and partiers.

Thankfully it was still early, and while there were predators about, none wanted to tangle with someone in spellarmor. I willed the mask to slither back into place, and considered my next option as I ambled out of the slums where we clung to our ragged existence.

A few figures lurked in the shadows, but none made any threatening motions as I passed. I kept a hand on Ariela anyway, though I didn't draw her. I didn't want anyone to feel threatened. I just wanted to be left alone.

My wish was granted, and a few minutes later I emerged into the safer part of town, which was unironically called the Buffer. It was the demarcation between the poor and worthless, and the upper echelon of society.

In the space of three city blocks you go from sludge-covered alleys and precariously stacked flops to wide, well lit streets patrolled by sweeper drones. Those do what they sound like and clean the streets, but they can also disintegrate undesirables when needed.

A clean white disk whizzed overhead, its lenses whirring as it scanned and identified me. Had it been unable to do so, then the local militia would be instantly alerted, and some of the scariest mercs in the sector would come have a little chat with me.

The drone gave a satisfied whir as it zoomed off to hassle the next person emerging from the flopstacks, and I hurried up the wide walkway, which contained a smattering of lower class service people trudging to jobs they hated.

The Buffer ended at a twenty-meter wall molded from blasteel, a magical blending of metal, plastic, and who knows what else. Bulky turrets dotted the wall at twenty-meter intervals, their barrels aimed into the Buffer as an ever-present reminder to mind our manners.

The trickle of traffic passed under a tall archway, with a pair of turrets turned in our direction as we flowed through. Apparently guards had been a liability, so they removed them—cheaper, and disgruntled workers can't really hold a turret hostage.

I passed through, tensing as the barrels swiveled in my direction. I passed whatever scan they were conducting, and finally exhaled the breath I'd been holding as I made it to the other side.

It was like entering a different world. Gone were all pollution, all garbage, all graphiti, and anyone who looked like they belonged in the stacks. The buildings were tall, white, and gleaming, and if they lacked the elegance and age of the academy they were still impressive.

The people allowed through were all presentable, at least enough to fit into a menial job. I didn't even have that much. What I did have was a price that I couldn't put off paying any longer. I made the first right past the checkpoint, and walked into the first building.

Arcan's Bonds was located where it was for a reason. The big purple magi-scrawl on the side of the wall was the first thing desperate people saw when crawling out of the gutter. *Get money NOW!* It was effective. Depths, that sign was how I'd originally met Arcan.

I hustled inside the building, and was unsurprised to find several people in line ahead of me. At least the place was chilled, an inexpensive *water* magic, but one that many shop owners skimped on in the stacks. Here though? Couldn't make the nice people hot, now could we? I wish I could afford to live here.

A tall, aging merc stood behind the counter, his bald pate reflecting the thin lights above. His scarlet cyber-eyes were as inhuman as ever, and they whirred as he focused on me.

"Jerek," Arcan's no-nonsense voice boomed from behind a wide counter. He rested two thick arms on the worn plastic, and stared hard at me. "I haven't heard from anyone on the *Remora*, but the number one pick for first casualty comes walking in. Give it to me straight, kid. What happened? Tell me you've got my money."

"Total wipe," I led with, which was how one talked to mercs. They're all battle stats and mission reports. "Lurkers. They took the ship, and I managed to sneak aboard the landing strut before they took off."

Arcan gave a derisive snort. "So you stowed back to Kemet on your own ship, with your tail between your legs?"

"As opposed to what?" I snapped, the weight of recent events finally cracking my composure. The same way our world was going to crack. "They'd already taken out our muscle and command. What do you think I could have done, Arcan? Please, enlighten me. Tell me how you would have played it."

Arcan eyed me curiously for a long time, and I couldn't tell if he was angry or confused, or both. His next words made it clear.

"I wouldn't have landed my sorry ass in the situation to begin with." Arcan's eyes narrowed, and he tugged on the end of his beard as if deciding whether or not I got to live. "I told you that trip was trouble. I told you there wasn't anything out there."

"But there was," I countered, unholstering the pistol I'd taken from the weapon's locker and placing it on the counter. I hadn't spent a lot of time with the sleek black weapon, but it had to be worth something. "I came back with a sidearm and a set of armor that predates planetfall by a *lot*. Listen. Take the pistol as collateral, and give me one day to bring the armor to the academy and get it appraised. I'm telling you...it's priceless. The armory will want this."

"Priceless doesn't pay my rent on this hole." Arcan folded those tree trunk arms, and his scowl deepened. "Your bond goes up 20% a day, and if you skip out on me I will hunt you down personally. I won't hire a merc. I'll do it myself, kid. I ran with your father for nearly three decades. We came up in the arena together. If he could see you wheeling right now it would break his heart. Assuming you ain't already broken it beyond repair. Shame. He deserved better."

That stung, especially given how long I'd known Arcan. Normally I'd have gotten even angrier, and maybe said some regretful things. It's funny how the impending dissolution of your planet can change your whole perspective.

"You're right," I agreed. Then I folded my arms to match

him. One of my instructors at the academy had said that mirroring body language made people nicer or something. "Here's the thing, Arcan. I need the armor. For at least a few days. I can't part with it. Let me be very clear about that. I'm walking out wearing this armor."

Arcan's eyes narrowed to slits and his voice went deathly quiet, barely audible over the hiss of cool air drifting down from the vent above. "You don't get to dictate terms here, kid."

"Yeah, I do." I wrestled hard with the anger. I knew my rights, and both the sidearm and the armor were mine. "You can't take them, and you know it."

"Are you really going to make me report you and send a tracer?" Arcan shook his head sadly. "I thought you were better than that, kid. You've never had a problem admitting when you were wrong before. Give me the armor. If it really is what you say it is then I'll see that you get 5% of the profit."

In my heart of hearts I wished I could disintegrate him where he stood, or do something equally impressive. What Arcan was doing? Tantamount to robbery in my book, and done often. In fact as I looked up and down the counter I saw three other people getting shaken down just like I was.

"No." I met Arcan's gaze without flinching. "Let me tell you how this is going to go. I get you, Arcan. I understand how my dad and his merc buddies think. You want credits. Always more credits. That's the bottom line. If you're not going to give me an extension, then I'll pay. But not with the armor."

I did something that might qualify as insane. It certainly qualified as risky, and maybe stupid. I withdrew Ariela from my holster and set her gently on the counter, then I gently spun her, and pushed her grip-first toward Arcan.

"You give me five thousand credits, and she's yours." I paused to let him survey the weapon, something he must remember from his time merc-ing with my father. "Keep three for the bond, then pay me out the rest."

"Kid, you get that this isn't collateral, right?" Arcan's eyes were wide now. Thick with disbelief. "If you do this, and your old man hears, I'm going to tell him I tried to talk you out of hawking your inheritance."

"That's the truth, and I'll back you up," I agreed, pushing the pistol a bit closer to him. "Five thousand credits is a joke for a fully realized eldimagus, and we both know it. Take the win, Arcan."

"Why are you doing this, kid?" Arcan's gaze had gone suspicious now, and he leaned closer to study me. "Do you really hate your dad this much? Is this a way to get back at him? Why do you need the money so bad? It can't be about the armor. I know you're into all that history stuff, but you've never much cared about weapons. Not like the rest of us."

I took a long, slow breath before answering. I needed him to go along with this, without immediately calling my father the instant I left the shop.

"Listen, Arcan. I get that you don't like me."

He gave a snort of agreement.

"This armor is important," I continued, trying to reach whatever part of him was still human. "Not just to me, or even to the academy. I have to get it to the right people, and I have to do it soon."

I considered telling him more, but I had no proof, and didn't really even have all the facts.

"Fine. Your loss." He scooped Ariela up lovingly in both hands, then ducked through the curtain separating the back room. Part of me wanted to follow, but I knew there was no way he'd double-cross me. Pawn brokers who did that sort of thing didn't live long.

I picked up the plain spellpistol I'd left on the counter, and slid it into Ariela's holster. The weight was off, and the fact that it couldn't fire slugs really bothered me. Ariela had saved my life more than once. What if I ran into a situation where I was out of spells?

Ah, well. I had to work with what I had, and firmly believed the armor really was that important. I needed to figure out how it worked, and how it knew what was going to happen to our world.

That made my next call even more uncomfortable than visiting Arcan.

9

A strange sense of resolve bolstered me as I left Arcan's pawn shop. I had two thousand and thirty-four credits on my chip, and my bond was paid off. That meant that for good or ill my destiny was now my own.

Until my father found out I'd sold Ariela, and my life was abruptly terminated. I figured that would happen sometime in the next few hours, when Arcan called him. That gave me the balance of the morning and maybe the afternoon to figure out what was going on with the hypothetical destruction of our planet.

I stood there on the corner of the busy boulevard, under the watchful eyes of circling sweeper drones, and tried to figure out what the smartest play was. I could try taking the armor to the academy. I'd been a pretty good student, and still knew some of the faculty. The armory staff would wet themselves to be the first to break the discovery of something this old.

Some might have contacts with the ministry, which was

where I'd need to ultimately end up. That would take time, though, and there was no guarantee of success.

There was a much, much faster way to get my case in front of the minister, but I was reluctant to use it, even with the fate of the world in the balance.

It meant calling my mother.

Now, I know what you're thinking. How bad can that be? Was she mean? No. My mother was nothing if not polite. Would she overly mother me? Nope. She expected me to make my own way in the world, and treated me like an equal most of the time.

So why was I so reluctant to call her? Because my mother was sleeping with the minister. Two years ago my mother, the then headmistress of the academy you hear me going on about, left my father...for our minister, the woman who runs our entire government.

My mom has always been type A, a real ambitious go-getter, and apparently back in the day so was my dad. They were the real power couple. After he retired from the arena, though, he lost his edge. Mom didn't. Her career went orbital, and she ended up running the entire academy while my father lived on subsistence.

That made him, and by extension me, my mom's embarrassing other life. The tether that she didn't want to be reminded of. I knew she loved me, but I also knew that she was embarrassed of her humble beginnings, and that a part of her would always resent me for it.

Whenever I called her, which I tried to avoid, it was almost always because I needed something. I carefully withdrew my comm, and looked around to make sure no one was watching me. Other than a sweeper drone no one paid me the slightest attention.

My comm vibrated as the connection resolved, then a

hologram of my mother's face sprang into existence over the device. The lines around her eyes had spread a little further, and I didn't recall ever having seen her look that tired.

"Hey, sweetie." She offered an exhausted smile. "Now is a really, really bad time. How much do you need? I don't need details, just a reason."

"Mom, I stumbled on something bad. Something you need to know about." There was so much I wanted to say to her as I stared down at the holo, wishing she were there in person. My mother was the smartest person I knew, and if anyone could solve this it was her. "The comet destabilized our orbit. The quakes are going to get worse, and our planet is coming apart. I don't know how long it will take. Days maybe? I figured if anyone knew about it, that it would be you guys and—"

"How did you know?" My mother's expression tightened, and her voice was flat. She glanced behind her, then back at the holo. "This is important, Jerek. How did you come upon this information? Who told you?"

I hesitated. I didn't know why, but something made me reluctant to tell her about the armor.

"Mom, why does that matter?" I evaded, playing for time. "Obviously from your reaction it's true. What the depths is going on? What is the ministry doing about it?"

"Stop." The word carried all the force of my mother's sternest voice, the one that had halted me in my tracks as a toddler. "Jerek, if they find out you know, if you try to go public, then they will take steps to silence you. They're trying to avoid a panic. Now tell me...how did you know?"

"I found something," I blurted. If I couldn't trust my mom, then who could I trust? "It's old. Lost tech, from early in the dragonflight's history, before the Vagrant Fleet splintered. That tech claims the comet was deliberately sent our way. Someone used *void* magic to fling a small moon at us."

My mom's sapphire eyes widened, and her mouth worked like a fish. I'd never seen her speechless. Not once. I didn't even think it was possible, but there it was.

"I'll get this information to the minister immediately, but she's going to want to talk to you in person." She leaned closer, her face growing a bit larger. "Jerek, you need to be careful. Grab a train and get here as soon as possible. Have you told anyone else about this?"

"Of course not." I left out Briff, as I saw no sense in involving the hatchling. The drone whirred by overhead again, and I tried not to ascribe anything sinister to its motives. "Mom, if the world is coming apart we need a ship. We need to get off."

Mom's mask, that careful professional facade she had so perfected, shattered. Her eyes were wet, and she wore her compassion openly. "If you get here I can get you a seat, honey. But you need to get here quick."

I went cold. "What about Dad?"

"There's nothing I can do for him." She shook her head sadly. "You have no idea how precious every seat is. They're talking about abandoning the armory because there simply aren't enough ships. We're saving the best and brightest. I will always treasure my time with your father, and we made something wonderful together, but he is neither of those things, Jer."

Conflicting emotions raged, all bad. I loved the academy, and the armory represented our people's history, and legacy, and wealth. Our pride. Losing it would break us as a people, and I hadn't even considered that it would happen when the world came apart. But that still wasn't the most important thing.

"I'm not leaving dad behind." I shook my head, and started moving up the street toward the closest tram terminal. They were everywhere here, and absolutely pristine to boot. Not at all like my neighborhood.

"You were always like this. Even as a child. I know you aren't going to relent. Hold on. I'm conferencing in your father." Her face moved to the side, her attention obviously on her own comm.

A moment later the hologram rippled, then split into two. The first was my mother, the second my father, seated on his hoverchair back in the flop.

"Do I even want to know?" He scrubbed his fingers through mussed hair. "What has he done this time, Irala?"

"Hello, Dag." There was affection in her voice, more than I'd expected. "It's not what he's done. It's what he won't do. Let's say, hypothetically speaking, that our world were about to end. Let's say that I ordered your son to come to me, because I could save him. He's refusing, because he wants to save you too. Something that is not within my power to do. Please tell your son not to be a sentimental fool."

My father stared adoringly at my mother, and it broke my heart. All the love was still there, though it lay beneath an oily residue of anger and resentment.

"Jerek," my father said, as if my mother hadn't spoken. "Why did you pawn Ariela?" His voice had gone deadly calm, which was never a good sign.

Suddenly I was glad it was a holo, instead of in person.

"It was that or give up the armor. Dad, Mom is right. Something bad is going down, and our world is coming apart. This armor might help me save people. I can't explain it any better than that. I'm sorry."

He kept a tight rein on his anger as he turned back to my

mom's holo, who'd remained silent during our exchange. "Our world is seriously ending? These quakes are that bad?"

"I'm afraid so. But you can't tell anyone, Dag. I mean that."

"You've got my bond," he offered, almost without thinking. To my father that was unbreakable, and my mother knew that better than anyone. "And you're telling me that Jerek won't take a free ticket off this rock?"

"Yeah," she said softly, her gaze locked onto him. "I'm sorry, Dag. I really am. I'd save you if I could, you know that."

"I know. You're not the minister, sweetie. You're just sleeping with her." My father delivered a rakish grin, and for just an instant was the godly gladiator I'd known in my childhood. He turned to me, and was suddenly crusty old dad again. "Jer, don't be an idiot. If you've got a ticket off this rock, then you take it. You let me stay behind and die heroically, so your mom can feel guilty about it."

My mom actually laughed at that, laughed like she'd used to. I found the whole exchange mortifying, but for them it seemed cathartic.

"Fine," I agreed, hating myself. My feet had already carried me to the tram terminal, though I hadn't selected a destination yet. "I will go to Mom. But only to show her and the minister this armor. I am not giving up."

"Of course not, sweetie," my mom said in a way that made it very clear I was absolutely giving up. She turned to my dad. "Die well, Dag."

He nodded at her, and left the holo. My mom disappeared a moment later.

I was left standing there, with not a lot of choices. I needed to get to my mom, on the northern continent. That meant a long tram ride, and plenty of time to think about how to handle things when I arrived.

A sort of numbness stole over me as I waved my hand over the scanner and tapped Thebes, the capital, as a destination. I filed past the security turrets and into the tram car, which was mercifully empty. I took a seat in one of the molded plastic seats, and then willed the helmet to slither into place.

It obliged, and the HUD lit as the tram lurched into motion. I was whisked along the track, the train gathering speed as we reached a main rail. I'd have about four hours to collect myself before I arrived, but I wasn't sure how to make best use of that time.

I could watch local news reports, but those would be heavily sanitized. I could try to learn more about the armor.

Or I could sleep.

Guess which one won out?

I woke about three hours later, per the tram's chronometer. I blinked blearily around trying to figure out what had woken me. A subsonic sound that I could feel as much as hear thrummed through me to the point of being physically painful.

A glance through the tram's windows at the mountains in the distance revealed the cause.

Something like rain, but in reverse. A cloud of tiny objects rose from the mountains, whipped up into a funnel that spun into the sky with incredible speed. The smattering became a torrent, and my jaw fell open as the mountain dissolved before my eyes, and was sucked up the funnel and into orbit.

The entire Sek mountain range, one of the largest in the world, was being ripped free of our world like so much dust.

As I watched, as the tram sped along, the phenomenon

spread. Smaller mountains, then foothills, and finally neighboring fields were torn from our world and sucked into the sky, just as the armored had warned.

Even inside the tram I could hear the awful noise, like the universe being torn in half. The wave of destruction rolled across the field, racing ever closer to the monorail as it obliterated everything in its path.

I backed into the tram's far wall, not that it would do any good. The unraveling burst upon us, and the monorail came apart in a screech of tortured metal. I was flung into the ceiling, then dashed into the floor, then into a window, which cracked but miraculously held.

It afforded a perfect view of the chaos around me. I watched helplessly as people, tram cars, the monorail, and the land beneath it all were violently hurled into the sky.

Then a hunk of monorail slammed into my tram car, and it exploded, tossing me into the storm of death, and up towards space.

10

I tumbled end over end, bouncing off debris and doing my best not to be crushed by the larger pieces of what had been a sprawling city just a few minutes ago. Up and up I went, thrust into the sky as gravity reversed on itself.

As I twisted around I saw where we were going... straight into the sun. Every bit of that debris had been torn loose by its much stronger gravity field. And I was part of that debris.

I spun back around, and my heart thundered when I saw how high I already was. I was out of the lower atmosphere, and it had happened in less than a minute. How fast was I going?

"It can't end like this." I held back a sob, though I wasn't sure who I was trying to impress. I gave in to panic for a good thirty seconds as the world fell further and further away from me.

My father's voice thundered in my head. *Survive. Find a way. Focus on what you can do.*

So I did.

"Okay," I muttered, wincing as I ricocheted off of a mail kiosk. "What can I control?"

The armor had surprised me time and again. Now my fate rested entirely in its figurative hands. If it had a miracle, maybe I could save myself. If not, well, at least I'd have an enjoyable view as I fell into the freaking sun.

When I'd needed a helmet I'd thought about it, and gotten one. You know what I needed right now? Thrusters. Or wings. Or something. I thought hard about momentum, and about getting back to the planet.

An intelligence answered within the armor, and seemed to be reaching for something in me. The only thing it could want was magic, so I fed it a sliver of *dream*. A discordant chime sounded in the helmet.

"Okay, wrong magic. Please don't tell me you need *void*, because I don't have it." I closed my eyes, and offered the only other type of magic I had. *Fire*.

A more friendly chime played, and the suit drew deeply from my magical reserves. A moment later flame burst from both boots and from both palms.

I'd like to tell you I gracefully assumed control, but, uh, it didn't really go down like that.

I cartwheeled wildly out of control, spinning first one way, and then another as I struggled in vain to control the thrust coming from all four of my limbs at the same time. It turns out that flying spellarmor is not a skill I possess. Who knew?

After a lot of fumbling I managed to dodge over a piece of concrete that looked like it had come from a monorail pylon, then fired a quick thrust from the right foot in an attempt to stabilize my flight.

It actually worked!

I flew in a more or less straight line for an entire three

meters, right up until I slammed into another tram car. The window cracked, but held. This car actually held people, but even as I called out to them I realized it was too late.

The passengers stared sightlessly ahead, dead of suffocation, or maybe exposure. But dead all the same.

I wasn't going to end up the same way.

I focused on flying, and kept practicing little bursts to get around hunks of debris. Instead of flying back to the planet I was trying to work my way to the outer edge of the cyclone streaming up from the surface.

Many harrowing minutes later I finally did exactly that, but by that time I reached the edge I'd left the atmosphere entirely. The planet lay below me, a spray of rock rising like droplets of water leaking from the sector's largest balloon.

Seeing it from this vantage was terrifying, and made it clear that the entire planet was in trouble. Several smaller leaks had appeared, all on the northern continent, the side closest to the sun.

I pressed my arms to my sides and dove toward the planet, pouring as much *fire* magic into the armor as I could muster. The armor picked up speed, and meter by agonizing meter I pulled myself closer.

The further I got from the debris field the easier flying became, and eventually the planet's gravity grabbed hold of me and started pulling me in. Apparently whatever the anomaly was it was localized to one area. If I could stay clear of that funnel I could make it back down.

I studied the affected part of the planet as I flew closer, and was relieved to see that the edge of the destruction stopped several hundred kilometers from dad's flop, and from the academy. He and Briff were okay for the moment, certainly in a less precarious position than I was.

I fed more *fire* to the armor, which was already becoming

a strain. *Fire* seemed wrong somehow, like it wasn't perfectly suited to the job and the armor was making do. Maybe that made the process more expensive, but whatever the reason I was running out of juice. Fast.

I pushed harder, and it started to burn. Literally. My shirt burst into flames over the heart as the suit eagerly drank the magic I fed it. The suit inched closer and closer to the planet until, suddenly, almost gently, we were seized by its gravity well and pulled down.

"WooHOO!" I bellowed, wrapping my arms tight against my body as the armor began re-entry. Somehow it looked like I might actually survive this.

The armor began to redden as we skimmed through the atmosphere, and the internal temperature rose to uncomfortable levels. Thankfully, one of the benefits of possessing *fire* magic is natural resistance to heat. What would cook a normal person kept me toasty warm as we descended.

Then, just like that, I was in free fall. Wind buffeted me about, but my momentum sliced through billowing clouds as I tumbled back toward Kemet.

Before long I could pick out cities, and used the thrusters to angle my flight closer to the stacks where my dad lived, which lay uncomfortably close to the flow of rock still streaming from the planet. I suspected that meant my dad's flop would be in the next area to go, and after that the academy itself.

I had to get him out. I mean, assuming I survived a fall from orbit.

My dilemma was now becoming clear. I was falling at terminal velocity toward my destination, and I'd used most of my magic making it this far. I could probably slow my momentum some as I got closer, but there was no way I was going to be able to stop myself.

I needed a soft landing. A liquid landing, ideally.

Unfortunately, there were no lakes within ten kilos of the sprawl around my dad's flop. There was, however, a sewage treatment plant no more than three clicks away. I grew up downwind of the smell, which taught me all about nausea.

I gave a heavy sigh as I stared down at the green speck that I guessed would be my probable destination. If this didn't work it would be an ignoble end. If it did work I would never get the armor clean again. But at least I'd be alive.

I pinned my arms to my sides, which was easier since I'd gotten stronger. I held them there, locking my elbows and angling the thrust downward.

Reaching deep was an understatement. As the city spun up at me, the flopstacks grasping at the sky like misshapen fingers, I poured everything I had into the armor.

Every bit of *fire* I could muster roared from my chest in a torrent of magical flame, washing into the armor and out the thrusters. But the armor was damned heavy, and inertia is one hell of a thing.

The flame from my hands and feet went blue, then white. The armor began to slow, but the lake of mucus-yellow sludge was rushing up at me far too quickly for me to stop.

"Oh, depths," I gasped, pushing even harder. If I came down too fast it wouldn't matter that I was hitting liquid. I'd still break every bone in my body.

The flow of magic intensified, and I reached deeper than I ever had, past the skin to the root of the magic itself. I'd always known that was possible, but I'd never been in a desperate enough situation to battle past the pain it caused.

Something cracked open inside me, and a fresh river of

flame poured into the armor. An answering chime came, and I shifted my focus from the pool of sludge to the paper doll in the corner of my HUD.

The trident icon was now lit, and I assume that's what the chime had been telling me.

I didn't have time to study it, and turned my attention back to maintaining thrust. I was slowing, but not nearly enough.

I slammed into the sludge in a tremendous geyser, and blackness took me as my head smacked into the helmet.

INTERLUDE II

Jolene waved a hand over her holodesk, one of the final models created before her exodus. The glassy surface shimmered, and the illusion tilted upwards slightly for ease of viewing.

The background was a sea of glittering stars, with the Erkadi Rift spinning slowly in the distance. She found its vibrant green clouds alluring, and they were a reminder that the Krox lurked within, now led by Frit. That made them enemies, as much as the Confederacy.

A missive, the spell equivalent of a comm call, blinked into existence on the center of the screen. She tapped the icon, a ghostly figure whispering into an ear, and Minister Ramachan's tired face filled the screen.

"Ah, Minister, what an unexpected pleasure." Jolene delivered her best smile, which wasn't hard given how much she was enjoying her imminent triumph. "Were there some final details to discuss before I depart the system?"

Ramachan's bloodless face stared back at Jolene, devoid of all humor and all compromise. She fixed Jolene with a martial stare, the kind befitting the leader of a mercenary world.

"You already know." Ramachan extended an accusatory finger, and her hand trembled as she stabbed it in Jolene's direction. "This whole thing was a ruse, wasn't it? A way to steal the fleet."

"Minister, this is hardly fair." Jolene leaned back in her chair, and adopted a reproving expression. "You haven't told me what this is in regards to. I understand my people have a somewhat deserved reputation for being canny trade partners, but the deal we struck is more than equitable—"

"It would be," Ramachan interrupted, "if you'd negotiated in good faith. Kemet's orbit has destabilized. I know you're aware. You were probably aware before I was. So I'm forced to ask myself, why would you feign ignorance? Those are the actions of a guilty conscience, one seeking plausible deniability."

Jolene gave a reluctant, exaggerated sigh. She raised a single perfect eyebrow, slowly. "You are testing my patience, Minister. I do not appreciate unsupported accusations. Do you have some evidence you'd like to present to back up your vague allegations? Yes, I have become aware of your planet's predicament, but that is hardly my fault. Besides," she said as she paused and offered a smile, "it is quite possible you might find a solution to this crisis. I don't want to assume that you won't, nor do I want to spook your populace by canceling the trade deal. Is that what you're telling me you'd like to do? Simply pay the cancellation fee, and I will have the trade moon diverted."

Ramachan's face went splotchy, and for a moment Jolene hoped she might actually start shouting. Instead, the woman gradually regained her composure, and did not speak until after she'd regained it fully.

"I have evidence that magic was used," the minister said. She leaned closer to the screen, and her eyes narrowed. "*Void* magic. It altered the course of the comet. That thing was aimed at our world, *Jolene*. Aimed by *you*, I'm willing to bet. I don't have evidence, but I will, eventually. And when I do you can bet that I will bring it to the Confederacy."

"If you make any such false allegations," Jolene replied softly, steepling her fingers as she peered over them at her adversary, "then I will also go to the Confederacy. Their courts take defamation quite seriously. Now I am very sorry for your local troubles, Minister, and I don't mind admitting that I do plan to profit off them. However, I am not the heartless monster you assume me to be. If you somehow avert this catastrophe, and satisfy your quota to the trade moon, then we make great profit and everyone wins. I wish you no ill will, Minister, but only a fool ignores an opportunity."

The minister's anger faltered, though her gaze was still clotted with suspicion. Her nostrils flared, but she said nothing for long moments.

"Very well," Ramachan finally said, her tone now controlled. "I will accept you at your word, until I have evidence. But make no mistake, Jolene. If you are responsible for this, then I will prove it, and I will see that you are taken down."

"Of course," Jolene agreed, stifling the small surge of fear that Ramachan might somehow make good on her threat. So far as Jolene knew, they had no way to communicate directly with the Confederacy, not through any official channels. That should buy her plenty of time.

"Good day." The missive ended, leaving Jolene with her thoughts.

She didn't like that her adversary suspected her, and it

alarmed her that someone possessed the magitech necessary to detect her involvement. What if they could somehow tie it back to her? After everything she'd seen, Jolene knew better than to assume she was safe.

Should she take further action?

No, that would only confirm the minister's suspicions. As difficult as it was, all she could do was sit back and wait.

If there was any silver lining it was that Ramachan would soon have much bigger problems to deal with.

11

_____

I woke up lying in the shallow end of the sludge lake, the armor mostly covered by viscous yellow goo. Thankfully the environmental seal was intact, insulating me from a wonderful aroma that I wasn't eager to get acquainted with.

What had woken me became clear when it poked me in the chest a second time. I leaned into a sitting position, and a trio of small humanoids scurried away as the leader dropped a long stick he'd been using to poke me.

At first I thought they were children, but if so these were the best armed ten-year-olds I'd ever run afoul of. Their scavenged combat armor was in good repair, and each had a pistol belted at their side. Small caliber, maybe, but enough for your average scav to worry about.

"Ey dere, fellow. Seem amite prickly." The lead figure trotted a bit closer. His voice was much deeper than I'd expected. "If yer gonna die, dafellows and I would appreciate it if you'd get on with it. Joost expire, alright, mate?"

I leaned back in the muck, instantly relieved. It was just

drifters. They could be dangerous, but nothing they could do was getting through my armor.

"Zat mean he expired?" One of the other drifters approached, and prodded me with a booted foot.

"No," I croaked, my throat raw for some reason. I took a deep breath and rolled over onto my side, then into a kneeling position. The drifters scurried backwards when I raised my hands. "I just got flung out of that."

I pointed shakily at the funnel cloud dominating the western horizon, the tornado of the gods, tearing rock, people, and everything else from that part of the world. Even this far away I could still hear that awful tearing sound.

"You joost came from that?" the third drifter asked, this one female. Her drawl was much easier to understand than the others. "This fooker is tougher than he looks. Come on, let's go. We're wastin' daylight."

The trio retreated down the shore of the sludge lake, and used their long sticks to prod the edge. I wondered what they found that made it worth the effort, then decided I really didn't want to know. The sludge came from all waste from the entire sprawl. Yuck.

I trudged up onto the shore, and started toward a random alleyway that led west. It might be a rat's nest, but it was my rat's nest and I knew it well. No one bothered me as I plodded by, though quite a few scavs cringed or winced as they walked past. It made me even more glad I couldn't smell myself.

The exhaustion made me want to close my eyes on the spot, but I knew if I did I'd never open them again. No self-respecting scav would pass up the opportunity to steal my armor, and the smart ones would sell my body to a chop shop to sweeten their payday.

No, I definitely couldn't fall asleep.

It took maybe ten minutes to wind my way back to my dad's flop, my first stop. I paused in the doorway, and leaned my head inside. "Dad? We need to talk. Right now."

"Are you depths-damned serious?" Dad came floating out on his hoverchair, a beer in one hand and the holo remote in the other. At least he was out of the recliner. "We *just* agreed that you were going to meet your mom. You can't save me, kid. Jer...wait, what happened to you? What is that SMELL?"

He finally seemed aware of my appearance, which in a word was...horrendous.

I didn't have time to catch him up. Every minute mattered now. Our world was on a timer. A short one. "Dad, my tram got sucked up into orbit. It's gone. The tram, the line, the city around it. All of it. Let that sink in."

He raised a skeptical eyebrow, which pissed me off. After everything I'd just gone through to survive...he didn't believe me?

"The whole city of Denalis is gone. The Sek mountains? Gone. You asked me why I hawked Ariela? Well, this armor just saved my life. Again. I clawed my way back down from orbit, and the sludge lake was the only available LZ. I'm damned lucky it was there. There's no reaching Mom, Dad. If we're going to survive, we're on our own."

My anger carried me through my little tirade, but as my father's expression hardened I lost a little steam. Skepticism and perceived disrespect warred across his face, and I prayed that common sense would win. My mom had told him this was real, and he trusted her implicitly, even now.

"I can let the Ariela thing go," he managed through gritted teeth, "but only if you live. If the world really is coming apart, then you need to get clear. Find a ship and get on it. ASAP. You can't afford to be saddled with a past-his-prime cripple."

I started to laugh. It rolled up out of me in waves, a release for all the pent-up tension, of the constant near-death escapes. After all this, my father was just going to stay home and die.

"You think this is funny?" my dad growled, his knuckles whitening around the beer.

"A little, yeah," I admitted. I almost took a step into the room before I remembered the sludge. "One of the most deadly shots in the sector just called himself useless. Dad, you are absolutely vital to the next part of my plan. I don't think I can survive without you, so, to use one of your favorite phrases, we don't have time for your pity party."

Now it was my dad's turn to laugh, which loosened something inside me. I hadn't been positive I could reach him.

"Your mother always warned me that one day you'd throw that phrase back in my face." He gave a lopsided grin, the same he'd delivered to my mother during the call. "Let's hear this terrible plan of yours."

"It's pretty bad." I shifted my weight, and wished I could lie down. Orbital re-entry had pushed me well past my limits, even with the armor's help. "It starts with you hosing me off. Once you aren't gagging any more we're heading to the pawn shop to get Ariela."

"And what," my dad interrupted, "makes you think that Arcan will part with her? He called just to taunt me about having her."

"Because I know where we can get a ship." Now it was my turn to smile, though my dad couldn't see my face under the armor. "We're going to need Arcan to outfit us, and we're going to need to pick up some muscle. Arcan will help with both, because he wants to survive the destruction of our planet and I can help him do that."

"Who do you have in mind for muscle? Can't let Arcan provide it all, or he'll gun us down the moment our backs are turned." My father's tone was dubious. He'd never had any faith in my friends.

"Briff." I raised a sludge-covered hand to forestall his protest. "I know you don't think he's worth much, but he's a crack shot, and he can get between us and a whole lot of nasty things I'd rather not have hit me in the face. We're going to need him to take the ship."

"Okay," my father allowed, tone still skeptical. "Let's say Briff pulls his weight. What ship are you planning to hit? Every vessel on this world is about to get damned popular."

That was the biggest failure point in my plan. I was gambling that the lurkers hadn't moved the *Remora*. I figured they didn't really have a reason to yet since word hadn't gotten out about the dissolution of our world.

If I could get there quickly enough the ship was probably still there. It would take weeks to scavenge her, and probably longer to find a buyer who'd take a ship with a wiped registration. She'd be guarded, of course, but I couldn't see them moving her.

"You let me worry about the ship," I finally said. "Finish your beer, and get your stuff. We're going to grab Briff first."

My father gave a shrug, then dropped his beer bottle into the bin with the others. "You know what? I'll go. Just to see how it plays out. Besides, if we somehow pull this off, your mother will have to live with the fact that I saved you."

I didn't point out that it was kind of the other way around. My dad wanted to have his last ride, and I didn't mind giving him that so long as he rode onto a ship and into orbit before this planet came apart.

As if to punctuate the thought the entire area began to shake. Not the swaying we'd had before, but a violent tremor that shook everything.

"Armor, can you estimate how long until this area is affected by the gravitational disturbance?" I tried to remember the term the armor had used. Geological instability? Hopefully it was smart enough to figure out what I meant.

A new feature blinked onto the HUD. A timer, counting down in draconic. I did the calculations in my head. The dragonflights had used a 365-day calendar broken into twelve lunar cycles, each 30 days long. The last five days of each year was called calibration, and was considered a time of rebirth.

Draconic civilization counted everything in relation to this calibration, and I swiftly converted it to our current calendar.

"We've got about six hours before this area is affected," I explained, as calmly as I could. "We need to get moving. Now."

I headed for Briff's without waiting for my dad, but was comforted when his hoverchair whirred along in my wake. Even with the constant quakes it didn't take long to reach Briff's. I wasn't a hundred percent sure he'd be home yet, but if the quake had knocked out his Quantum then there was no reason for him not to come back to his flop.

His door was open, as usual, and I poked my head in. The entire building shook, and I knew it was only going to get worse.

"Hey, Briff, you back?" I scanned his flop, and found him sitting on his couch, his wings raised to stabilize him against the shaking. His holo had vibrated off the stand onto the warped floor, and cans were jumping about on his floor making a bunch of tinny chimes.

"What the depths is this, Jer?" Briff struggled to rise, and eventually found his footing. "Why isn't it stopping?"

"This isn't an earthquake," I explained. "Grab your gear. We need to get out of here. Now."

My father zoomed up into the doorway and delivered his trademark judgmental stare. "You seriously have no idea what's going on? Have you not been following holo? It's all over everything."

"I was playing arena…" Briff gave an apologetic shrug. "So where are we going? And why is your dad with us?"

"The planet is coming apart." I glanced over my shoulder. The shaking was getting worse, and people were emerging from their flops and looking around. Panic would be the next stage. "We need to get ahead of this. I know where we can get a ship, but we're going to have to take it from some lurkers."

"Oh." Briff blinked at me with those unreadable slitted eyes. "Okay. Let's go then." He reached over and hefted his security guard breastplate, then affixed his pack to the back of it. "Do we have time to grab something to eat? I just got home and my fridge is empty."

"Is he even serious?" my father snarled.

"Dad." I put up a hand to forestall him. Mediating disputes between the two of them was going to be so much fun. "Briff, grab whatever food you have, because no, we don't have time to stop."

Briff's tail drooped, and he licked his fangs nervously. "I, uh, just ran out of algae. I was going to go to the store around lunch time."

"So you have no rations." My dad zoomed out of the flop.

"Come on, Jer. We don't need this riffraff. I'd rather take my chances with Arcan's mercs."

"Dad!" I snapped, rounding on him. "This is my op. You want to come along, awesome. But I'm calling the shots. Briff comes. We need him. You've never seen him fight, and you're just judging him by his appearance."

"Dragons should not be plump." My father stabbed a finger at Briff's gut, which to be fair was perhaps a bit on the larger side. "When was the last time you even flew? Can you even fly?"

"This is getting us nowhere," I growled, then turned back to Briff. "We'll see if Arcan can supply rations. If not, the lurkers may have some. Either way we don't have time to deal with it. In six hours this city is dust. Let's move."

12

I raised my arms, exposing the armor to the torrent of water spraying from the hose Briff held. The hatchling methodically removed the yellow sludge coating my suit, and I couldn't help but stare at the readout next to the paywater reservoir where the water was coming from. We were being charged both by the minute and by the liter. I had credits, thanks to Arcan, but it was still hard watching my account drain.

Instead, I focused on more interesting things, namely the armor's HUD. The trident icon above the paper doll had lit when I'd poured the *fire* magic into the armor during my frantic post-orbital adventure. At the time I hadn't noticed that a new icon had also appeared, this one an eye inside a triangle, greyed out just like the trident and crown had been.

The trident probably indicated some sort of weapons system, which I'd guess was connected to projecting energy from the suit's limbs. I'd have to study it when I found something to shoot at. The eye though? That symbology was all over ancient dragonflight tech, though not in this archaic form.

It symbolized divination magic, the very magic I was trained to use. I didn't yet know what the symbol would unlock, but I was damned excited to find out. Whatever it was might be tailored to my particular set of skills, and if ever there was a time I needed an edge it was now.

"So, Jerek," Briff rumbled, waving the hose to drench the back of the suit's legs. "I know we kind of glossed over this before, but you said the world's ending. Right? Whole thing is gonna blow up?"

"Pretty much," I affirmed, twisting the armor to provide a better target.

"Then why are we standing around hosing you off? I mean, shouldn't we be running for our lives?" Briff finished his work, and replaced the hose in the receptacle as I stood there dripping.

He'd done a fine job and a cursory examination revealed no remaining sludge, but the bath had cost two hundred and nineteen credits. Ouch. Over 10% of my funds just to clean some armor.

My dad bobbed a bit closer on his hoverchair, and delivered a pitying look to Briff. "You want me to explain it, Jer?"

"No." I knew my father would be an ass about it, and Briff was stressed enough. I needed him calm for what was to come. "Briff, we're heading through the security checkpoint. They'll never let us in if I'm covered in that goop, so we took a few minutes to fix that. Now we need to get moving. We've got a little over five hours to get this done. Try to look like you belong. Remember, you're muscle. Act like it. Just like back at school, you're the heavy bringing up the rear."

"You got it, Jer." Briff straightened, towering over me,

especially if you counted the wings jutting over his shoulders.

He might not be intimidating for a dragon, but the base level was pretty terrifying from my perspective. Add in a spellcannon, or even a conventional railgun, and he'd be properly menacing.

I took point, which felt odd, but since this was my op, that was where I belonged. My dad's hoverchair whirred behind me, and Briff brought up the rear. We didn't talk as we walked, thankfully. Nervous chatter wasn't a distraction I could really deal with right now.

As I retraced my steps to Arcan's pawn shop, I considered my impending plan. Theoretically the ship had four defenders. Two I'd seen, and two more that the guard had yelled out to. Add in a hypothetical two new arrivals and we were looking at something like six defenders. I seriously doubted it was more.

We'd need to disable the defenders, and we'd have the advantage of surprise if we played it right. Unfortunately, even if the initial assault went well, we were still looking at a room by room clear of the ship.

That might have been fun back when we were using paint pellets at the academy, but this would be very real, and very lethal. I still remember the void bolt that woman had hit me with. My armor might block a shot or two, but it didn't make me invincible.

We finally reached the gates leading through the buffer, which were clogged with people trying to get through. Most stood at a semicircle just outside the scanners, and for good reason.

They had no lawful business in the next sector, and the guns would cheerfully cut down anyone unauthorized who tried to enter. Blam, blam, blam...have a nice day, citizen.

Every now and then a maintenance worker would dart forward and slip through the turrets and drones, but most personnel were already on shift. That made it easy to pass through the crowd, who muttered darkly in our direction as we strode through their ranks.

"Yeah, that's right," my father boomed. "We've got commerce to be about. Get out of the way, scavs." His grin had a note of cruelty to it, a bit of the resentment he'd built for his neighbors leaking through.

"Excuse me," I said, stepping to the side to allow an old woman pushing a cart full of wilted mushrooms to pass. Most other people got out of my way, and I reached the edge of the crowd.

The precious minutes on the walk here had been useful for thinking, but now it was go time. I needed to convince Arcan, a hostile and shrewd negotiator, to make a deal based entirely on faith.

I didn't even tense as I passed beneath the checkpoint's watchful turrets, as for once I had more pressing concerns. My father followed on my heels, but when I glanced behind me I saw Briff frozen in place, his head swiveling from one turret to the next.

"I'm, ah, not usually allowed out unless I'm on shift." The hatchling took a step forward, and the scanners focused on him. His voice had risen a half octave when he spoke next. "They're going to let me through, right?"

The scanner winked green, and a visibly relieved Briff hurried through, his belly bouncing and tail swaying as he lumbered past the turrets. Ironically, he was far more likely to survive them than a human.

"This way." I swiftly made my way around the corner to Arcan's shop, but slowed when I saw it. The shop's front had two large windows, like most shops, and they afforded an excellent view of the crowd within.

The most people I'd ever seen had been maybe a dozen. There might be fifty people now, all being waited on by the three men at the counter. Those waiting held everything from spellcannons to refrigeration units, all aiming to get a little capital.

"Guess word's already gotten out," my dad groused, zooming a bit closer to the door.

"Not yet," I disagreed. "These are the smart people who are putting the pieces together. It's going to get a lot worse." I stepped in front of the pawn shop's scanner and the door slid open, allowing me to join the back of the line. I pitched my next words low, though they were covered by the hum of conversation in the room. "If they make an official state-ment, everyone is going to stampede for the safer parts of the planet. We need to be quick, before word gets out."

I shifted from foot to foot, but a grey-scaled hatchling with metal-tipped wings stood a few places ahead of me, effectively blocking my view. This was going to take hours, and when you were counting the survival of the planet in the double digits, every hour mattered.

"I ain't good for much, but I can take care of this." My father adopted a grim expression as his hoverchair whirred higher into the air. "I'm gonna have to eat a giant loaf of humble bread, so you kids had best appreciate this."

At first I wasn't sure what my dad meant. He'd drifted high enough that his head nearly bumped the track lights, making him visible to Arcan and his minions even with this large of a crowd.

"Well, if it isn't Dag the Slayer," Arcan's voice boomed through the room, smothering nearly every conversation. "Everyone get a good look. We've got a bonafide arena champion here, folks. Three years running, if you can believe that. Course, you might also notice that he's a bit shorter than he used to be. Looks like he's missing a couple legs. Why don't you tell us how you lost those, Dag?"

My father did something I didn't believe him capable of. He took the hit for the team, and he did it with grace.

"Yeah, sure, Arcan. You want my dignity? You can have it, as long as you hear out my boy right after." My dad gave a pained nod, the lines tightening around his eyes. He licked his lips, and seemed to force the words out. "Once upon a time I was a damned good arena captain. I can direct a squad. I'm a crack shot, one of the best in my day. I had the body. I had the reflexes. I had the magic."

Arcan gave an irritated snort, but didn't interrupt.

"Then I got arrogant," my father continued, his gaze now locked with Arcan's. "I ain't gettin' any younger, and I knew I couldn't run arena forever. I thought I could transition to a mercenary commander. Figured running five squads couldn't be that much harder than running one, so I recruited Arcan here and three other captains. Our very first job was down near New Cairo. Corporate dispute. They needed us to dip in, wipe out some research, and then get out. I chartered a dropship and everything. We infiltrated using orbital pods, like a damned holo."

"You told us it would be simple," Arcan snarled, his eyes narrowed. The hatchling in front of me had moved, and I saw the broker's fist tighten around Ariela's grip where she was belted around his hip. "Good money, you said. Better because we were only splitting it twenty-five ways, instead of the hundred and twenty-five the job called for. But you were a crap leader, Dag. You gave us no idea what we were walking into."

"You're right." My dad's spine went ramrod straight atop

his hoverchair, his posture every inch the doomed soldier facing the firing squad. "During the evac I stepped on a swarmer mine, and the nanites ate their way up to my thighs before they ran out of steam. After I went down I had no second designated, and we broke into five independent squads. Less than half of us made it out, and that was my fault."

"At least you're willing to own up to it. Only took you eleven years." Arcan slowly shook his head, then moved to the opening in the bar. "Your kid's got business, old man? Follow me. And expect me to apply an asshole surcharge to whatever you have in mind."

13

M y dad's hoverchair whirred through the crowd, which reacted much differently than I'd expected. It started slowly, at first, but quickly rippled through to the people at the edges.

They were saluting him.

Dag the Slayer rode proudly through that crowd, the adulation strengthening him the way sunlight straightened longgrass. A fair number were old enough to remember when my dad had been on top, and those who weren't recognized a man who'd just faced the depths and passed through them back into the light.

I trailed in his wake, unnoticed, with Briff dutifully bringing up the rear. I noted that his eyes ceaselessly scanned the crowd, the way a proper rear guard should. Pity my dad didn't see it.

We followed Arcan into his back room, a place we'd caught glimpses of but had never been allowed to enter. A pair of comfortable hovercouches, their leather cracked and well used, but clean, bobbed up and down opposite each other, a large table set between them.

That table had been forged from scrap metal, a panel from the outside of a frigate. It was at odds with the trophies lining the walls, ancient armor, or spellblades, and even a bulky G-141, one of the very earliest handheld railguns. I sensed a story there.

Arcan plopped down on one of the couches, which sagged much more than it should have. I chalked that up to cybernetic implants. Arcan was probably as much machine as man, though beyond his cyber-eyes none of those augmentations were obvious.

"Don't make yourself comfortable. You aren't staying." Arcan eyed my dad coldly, then shifted that heavy stare to me. "I'll honor my deal with your old man, but that doesn't mean I have to go along with whatever crazy scheme you're here for. Ariela is mine. I'm not parting with her. Consider her penance, Dag. And for depths sakes look me in the eye when you talk to me, kid."

"All right," I said, willing the helmet to slither back into the armor. I waited until the process completed before speaking. To my surprise I had no trouble meeting his gaze. "You're aware of the funnel going on northwest of here?"

Arcan gave an almost imperceptible nod. "There are three more now. News is wondering if a fifth will pop up soon. They still have no idea what's causing it."

"I do. And so does the ministry." I strode over to the hovercouch, and peered down at him with as much confidence as I could muster. If I failed here, more than my life was at stake. "That comet destabilized our orbit. Our planet is drifting closer to the sun, and the gravitational pressure is literally tearing our planet apart. We have days. Maybe less."

Arcan's only response was to lick his lips. He said nothing, just stared up at me from the couch.

"That doesn't concern you?" I finally asked.

"Oh, it does." Arcan folded well muscled arms, each crisscrossed with scars. "I still haven't heard a question though, or anything about business."

"I can get us a ship," I explained. I did my utmost to sound like a confident leader, though I'm not much of an actor. "It's not heavily guarded, and if we come in fast and hot we can take it."

"You know where the *Remora* is?" Arcan sat up in the couch, his interest apparent. "All right, kid. You have my attention."

"I know where it is," I agreed, elated that I had his interest. "I rode it back, and got a good look at the lurkers holding it. It wasn't heavily defended, and there's no way they've had a chance to sell it."

"Probably not," Arcan allowed, relaxing into his couch as he resumed his shrewd business man exterior. "But they might have moved it. Or escaped with it."

I shook my head. I'd considered both options, and neither was likely. "Moving it takes fuel, and requires a second secure location. It requires crew, and worst of all...it can attract attention. These people are lurkers. They're trying to fly under the scanner."

"But they *do* want to live," Arcan pointed out, giving a triumphant half smile. "And that means the ship could be gone, which makes your intel suspect at best."

He had me there, and I hesitated as I struggled to find a way forward.

My dad barked a short laugh, drawing everyone's attention. He delivered that crooked smile, the champion smile, to Arcan. "It's a better bet than the one I gave you. We all know you want to live, and while you've put away a few credits, I know you, Arcan. You don't own a ship. Everything you own is about to go kaput, unless you find a way off this rock. Berths are about to get real pricy, I think."

"Maybe," Arcan allowed, though his expression didn't yield any ground. "Let's say I'm interested in this intel. What outrageous cost do you have in mind?"

"We're going to have to take the ship from a squad of lurkers," I explained, folding my arms in imitation of him. To my surprise I felt the muscles. It felt good. We could do this. "They have no idea we're coming, and I want to maximize that advantage. I need you, and one other heavy to round out our squad."

"Squad?" Arcan barked a cruel laugh, the same kind I heard from my father on occasion. "You lot are not a squad. You've got a cripple, a fat dragon, and a scrawny fast-talking kid. Even if I brought the best heavy in the business it wouldn't make up for you lot."

I glanced at my father, expecting him to come to our defense. Instead he merely watched me expectantly, as he should have, I realized. I was the squad leader. It was my job to deal with stuff like this.

"I wasn't finished," I continued, meeting Arcan's gaze without flinching, something I was quite proud of. Resisting the urge to look away wasn't easy. "You're going to outfit us. Briff needs a railgun, and we aren't picky about what it is. Dad is going to be wielding Ariela, and you're giving him a suit of NTM environmental armor, something we can customize. You might think we're trash, but we are also your only hope of getting off this rock. Besides, if we're as bad as you think, then after we take the ship you can just mutiny and take over, right?"

No one laughed at that, though I'd meant it as a joke.

"I'm not giving up Ariela." Arcan rose to his feet, and now loomed over me. "I'm also not giving that waste of scales a railgun. Here's what I *will* do...I'll give your dad some armor, and a bottom of the line spellpistol. Something in need of maintenance. Your dragon can carry my G-141, and has my permission to gun down anything that attacks us. When we reach the ship he gives me my gun back. I will also provide a transport that will get us to the site where the *Remora* is stationed, and I will provide a real heavy, armed to the teeth."

"Wait a tick." I forced a deep breath before speaking, because what I wanted to say would definitely end any chance we had at a deal. Instead, I aimed for reasonable. "So if I understand what you're saying, you'll give us one rusty pistol and one suit of basic armor. Then, when we reach the ship, we are unarmed against this heavy you're bringing."

"Yeah, that's the general idea." I didn't at all enjoy Arcan's smile. "I can call her in right now. I know just the gal. Loyal. Deadly. And a survivor."

"So here's the compromise," I offered, knowing I'd have to give some ground. "You keep Ariela. That was my mistake, and you profited from it. But you meet the rest of the terms. You give my father and Briff the best weapons and armor available. You want this to succeed, right?"

He hesitated and I realized I'd found the leverage I needed. Arcan was a survivor too, which was why he valued it so much in whoever this heavy was.

"All right, you've got a deal." He rested a hand on Ariela's hilt, a jab at my father, and extended the other one to me.

I accepted the handshake, and he made a point of trying to crush my hand. I was shocked to realize I could return the grip, and did so. His eyes widened in an incredibly gratifying way.

"Partners," I said. "Make no mistake though, Arcan. I'm calling the shots on this op."

Arcan gave an approving nod. "Your kid's got balls, Dag."

"And I'm guessing your heavy is *your* kid?" my dad answered, his tone neutral.

I'd never heard of Arcan having a daughter, and my dad had never mentioned it. I wondered why.

"Yeah," Arcan agreed. He hurried to the back of the room, where another door stood behind a shelf. It wasn't exactly secret, but it would be easily missed by anyone glancing into the room. "Come on. Let's get loaded up, then I'll introduce you to Rava. We'll take her rover. How far away is this place?"

"About six hours," I grudgingly offered. He might be acting more friendly now that we'd made a deal, but Arcan stabbing us in the back wasn't a matter of if.

It was a matter of when.

14

One of the most important parts of leadership seemed to be jumping before everyone else jumped, so I started for the back door like I had some idea what I was doing. That prompted Arcan into motion, and the cybered merc led us through, into his storage bay.

We descended a short flight of metal stairs, and rows of floodlights came on one by one as we entered the room. The walls were lined with gun cages, all filled with various weaponry and ordnance.

Two six-wheeled rovers were parked next to each other, both battered, but in good repair. Each had the same matte black armor, which protected the cargo compartment in the rear of the vehicle.

Gun slits lined all sides so that defenders could rotate to any point quickly, but they were too small to allow a grenade or micro-mine to be tossed through.

One of the vehicles had an edge, though. A turret with a two-meter barrel was affixed to the top, and could be safely fired without exposing any of the crew. As expected, that was the one Arcan made for.

As he approached, I spotted movement at the far end of the room, against the concrete wall. A woman in black leather pants and a matching jacket had her feet propped up on a crate, while she lounged back in her chair.

Her attention was fixed on the holodisplay before her, the 3D images simulating the same combat arena I'd seen back at Briff's. She played the team's heavy, which meant she was in the rear.

To my mild surprise, her character raised her spell-cannon and lobbed a holographic ball of flame at an apparently empty spot. Just before the flame hit, an enemy scout moved into that position, and the fireball detonated all over their faceplate.

The scout flickered, then disappeared from the match.

"K-k-k-k-killing blow!" echoed throughout the room, the volume explaining why the woman hadn't realized we were here yet.

Arcan raised his wrist and tapped the controls on a sensor-bracelet. The holodisplay winked off, leaving the woman staring at empty space.

"Do you have any idea what you just ruined?" She shot to her feet, and stalked several steps closer to Arcan, short raven locks bobbing on her shoulders as she moved...moved like a cat. In a way that suggested cybernetic enhancement. "I was about to win the quarterfinals. The prize—"

"Our planet won't be here next week," Arcan snapped. He met his daughter's glare kilo for kilo, then jerked a thumb at the rover with the turret. "We're taking Betsy, and making a run for a ship before this whole planet shakes itself apart. Gear up, and zip the lip, kid."

"That's it?" she growled as her eyes narrowed. Leather

creaked as her hand wrapped around a spellpistol very similar to Ariela. "No explanation, just let's go?"

I was mostly fixated on the scene, but an amused snort from my dad drew my attention. He was staring at the woman in...pride? The kind of pride I'd always hoped he'd level in my direction. I raised an eyebrow, trying to understand.

Who was she?

"Okay, fine." Arcan's expression didn't offer her a millimeter. "Everyone else, the mouthy one here is my daughter, Rava. Rava, this is everyone. Rava is going to drive the rover to the *Remora*'s LZ, then gun down the opposition so we can escape this planet before it blows."

"Glad to have you," I found myself saying. I took a step closer and offered a hand. "My name's Jerek, and this is my op."

"Your op?" She blinked at me in genuine surprise, which softened her expression and highlighted clear brown eyes. The same color as my eyes. And my dad's. That was common enough not to occasion comment, but it still had me wondering.

"Yeah," Arcan reluctantly agreed. "Kid has intel on the ship, so we've agreed to give him lead until the ship is secured."

"All the same to me." Rava offered a nonchalant shrug. "Just let me grab my holounit." She waved a hand in the vague direction of Briff and me. "Either of you play? Single player is super boring, and I have a feeling Quantum is going to go down when the planet blows up."

"Uh," Briff managed, his wings fluffing nervously behind him. "Yeah, I play. Looks like you run as a heavy though, and that's the only role I know."

"That's all right." Rava delivered a crooked smile that

made my heart sink, because I'd just seen it...on my dad's face. "I can switch it up. I'm good at all roles."

I caught my dad's attention, pointed at Rava, and glared.

My dad whirred a little closer and shook his head. "Later. Now is not the time. Say nothing. Arcan doesn't know. Neither does your mom, for that matter."

I kept my mouth shut, but inside I couldn't disagree more strongly. Arcan's hatred of my father seemed a little too intense for a botched op that had happened decades ago. No, this was a personal kind of hatred, and now I understood exactly what had caused it.

"Briff, take the turret," I ordered as Arcan opened the rover's rear door. "Dad, Arcan, you're in back. Rava, I'll ride shotgun."

I'd often wondered at the origin of the term "ride shotgun". A shotgun had the worst range and accuracy out of any weapon I'd used, and was the very last gun I'd want while firing out a passenger window.

I moved around to the rover's side, and climbed into the navigator's seat next to Rava. She buckled into her harness with the efficiency of long practice, and fired up the rover's fusion reactor.

It was less efficient than *fire* magic, but since neither she nor her father were magically active, it was their only option.

The rover lurched into motion, all six tires hugging the concrete as the metal gate rolled up into the ceiling at our approach. We passed under it, then out onto the main road outside Arcan's shop.

The panic hadn't spread to much of the populace, at least that I could see. Traffic *was* beginning to thicken, though. And the sky had had grown awfully dark, despite the early hour.

"This is going to take forever," I muttered as I stared at the line of transports clogging both the street and the ramp leading onto the public freeway.

Rava calmly opened a compartment behind her chair and withdrew a pair of sunglasses, which hummed with electronics as she perched them on the bridge of her nose. "So where is this place, exactly?"

I considered my answer carefully. If I told her, I was giving up leverage. I decided trust was more important. "West of New Cairo, about a dozen clicks."

She nodded, and delivered another one of my father's smiles. Her feet engaged the pedals, and the vehicle leapt into motion. Only...not toward the road.

We bounced up over the curb, and into a trash-laden field that had accumulated at the base of the monorail. Rava expertly navigated around a wing fragment, then over the remains of a mech arm as we entered the scrapyard.

I held on for dear life as the rover tilted into angles that I was sure would cause us to topple. They never did.

"Inertia." Rava gave a delighted laugh next to us. "You're wondering how I can take these slopes, right?"

"Erk," was all I could manage as we went down a steep cliff toward a boulder field below.

Rava suddenly accelerated, and the wheels clung to the rock face as we shot down the hillside. She jerked up with a whoop as we hit the boulder fields, and I tasted blood as I accidentally bit my tongue.

We shot along at top speed, racing alongside the traffic on the freeway above us.

"You know what, Rava?" I asked, smiling up at the traffic we weren't in. "It's really nice to meet you."

"Whatever you say, kid." She gave a whoop as she accelerated again, loving the thrill in the same way my father did.

15

Most of the drive with Rava passed in silence. After the first few kilometers she was able to find an onramp that wasn't clogged, and we got out ahead of the crowds.

We hummed along, passing the exact same way I'd so recently come, but in reverse. This time I had a much better idea of what was going on, and much clearer goals.

Among them was learning more about the armor, which I'd been avoiding because I'd had more pressing things to deal with. Now I could tinker with it guilt free, knowing there was nothing else in the world I should be focusing on.

"Don't mind me if I start muttering to myself," I explained to Rava as I finally broke the silence. "I'm going to test a few things on my suit."

"Yeah, I was going to ask you about that." Rava tapped the autopilot button, then shifted in her seat to face me.

The way she moved made me absolutely positive she could snap my neck before I could draw my pistol. My new muscles suddenly felt a whole lot less impressive beside her cyberware.

"I've never seen that make," Rava continued. She touched my shoulder. "This polymer isn't in use anywhere I've seen. Where did you get it?"

"On a dreadnought." I flinched back from her, though I couldn't tell you why. I forced myself to relax, though I did notice her raised eyebrow. "It's at least seventy millennia old, and it has some sort of magical intelligence. I haven't figured out how to tap into it yet, but hopefully by the time we get there I'll have a better idea."

"Okay, Cap." Rava put her feet up on the dash. "I'm going to catch some zzz's. Happy muttering." She rested her head against the seat, and I kid you not, she started snoring instantly. I was genuinely impressed.

"Well, here goes. Okay, armor, are you capable of voice communication? If so, please activate that now, and utilize the language I am speaking in."

My helmet flowed into place of its own accord, surprising me, but I forced myself to remain calm and waited for the armor to finish whatever it was doing. The HUD lit, and a console appeared, the same one where I read text missives.

After a several second delay, text began to appear, writing itself in galactic standard for the first time.

I am capable of voice communication; however, magnetic interference prevents me from manifesting this ability.

I began to tremble. How could I not? This level of communication was far beyond what a piece of magitech should be capable of. This thing was fully sentient.

"Okay, how can I remove the interference?" I set my hands on my knees, and forced myself to sit still as I awaited an answer.

Either enhance the suit's transmission, remove the interference, or shorten the distance between us.

That gave me pause. "There is no distance between us, is there? You are the armor, right?"

No. I am linked to every Heka Aten suit, but I do not reside in any of them. I am currently in communication with three pilots.

That prompted about a million more questions, but I knew I needed a focused line of questions. One that led to us getting off this planet.

"Okay," I reasoned aloud. "Do you reside on the ship where I found the armor?"

Yes.

"I really wish you wouldn't talk so much." The magical intelligence apparently had no sense of humor, or maybe the joke was just bad. "So if you're on the ship, do you have access to the orbital scanners?"

That seemed like a long shot, but hey, why not try?

Yes. Would you like me to initiate a scan?

"Do that. Scan the following coordinates." I fed in the location where I'd escaped the *Remora*. "I want to confirm that a ship is still parked there. Can you do that?"

A hologram sprung up in my field of view, and it showed a top-down view of the site where I'd seen the lurkers. The *Remora* was still parked there, as were two rovers. I could see several figures walking around.

"I can't believe this is real time." I studied the figures. None wore the same armor I had anymore. All were in the battered lurker gear I'd seen on the others. "I don't suppose you can nuke them from orbit?"

Weapons offline. Even were they not, firing would liquify the surrounding area, and the target vessel would be destroyed.

Maybe I was imagining the sarcasm. Okay, so the ship couldn't help directly, but at the very least it could provide up-to-the-minute detail.

Then it hit me. I sat up straight, grinning. "Can you

run some sort of thermal scan? Or use *life* magic or something? I want to know how many lifeforms are inside that ship."

The hologram went translucent, exposing a cutaway view of the *Remora*. I counted six figures inside, plus four more around the compound. Yikes. But at least I had a head count.

By my estimates we had another four hours before we arrived, and now that I had a good idea of the defenders' attitude, I could start planning. If we did this fast and clean, we might be able to get in and seal the ship without dealing with the four people outside.

That still meant we were outnumbered, but that was where the concept of action economy came in. If five of us ran into a room and shot the first two lurkers, we could overwhelm them, and they'd only get two shots back. Divide and conquer, basically.

If it worked.

How would I be able to manage that, though? Briff wasn't exactly stealthy, and neither was my dad. They were going to see us coming unless I came up with a way to mitigate that.

I spent some time watching the figures inside the ship, trying to figure out who they were and what they might do based on nothing but their movements. It was just as maddening as you can imagine, at first anyway.

I quickly realized that two of the figures weren't moving very much at all. They stayed in the same places, never moving more than a meter or two. At first I'd thought they were third shift and just getting rest, but both figures got up and moved around their quarters regularly. They just never left them.

I called up a schematic of the *Remora*, which I hadn't

known that well, and referenced the area where they were located.

"Drakkon's frosty balls," I whispered. "They're in the brig!"

If I was right, it meant that we only had four people to contend with. It was even possible the pair in the brig might be allies, depending on why they were being held.

Now all I needed was a way for us to approach. I figured I had several hours to think about it, and then maybe I'd finally be able to impress my father and save our collective asses.

INTERLUDE III

J olene settled gracefully into the hovercouch's luxurious leather, one of the finest Shayan models, and waved a hand at the floating pitcher that bobbed up and down near it. The vessel drifted over and tilted to fill her goblet with scarlet lifewine, also the Shayan variety.

At one time such luxury had brought her comfort, but all that had been stripped when Skare had provided her first taste of the Blood of Nefarius. It had brought her power. Immense power. But also an endless thirst for more.

That insatiable need had driven her to terrible acts, and had blinded her to the situation until she'd nearly lost everything. She had regained control of herself, though truth be told, that was only because there was no source for the blood.

If Talifax showed up today—something she prayed daily would never occur—and offered her another taste, would she have the strength to decline? She doubted it. Her resolve would break and she would once more be a puppet.

Yet each day ended, and he did not return. That didn't mean he wouldn't. Time was fluid to a being like that.

That was one more reason why she needed to flee this sector forever. She needed to be away from enemies and temptations both, but she would do it on her terms. She might even reclaim a bit of her glory.

Booted footsteps rang in the hallway outside her sitting chamber, part of sprawling apartments deep within her flagship. Every bit of the decor had been designed with impressing guests in mind, and while she couldn't see the faces of the trio of armored men, she did note the long slow looks as their helmets panned around her chambers

"Welcome, War Leader Bortel." Jolene gestured, and hovercouches moved to each of her three guests.

Bortel, the tallest figure and the one in the lead, glanced at the couch, then back at her. His armor was pristine, and she doubted it had ever seen battle. "I'd just as soon conduct our business and return to my ship. Every moment I am here the risk of discovery grows."

"You are too cautious." Jolene raised a delicate eyebrow, and leaned a bit closer. "Everything has proceeded exactly as I said it would. We've already lived up to our part of the agreement."

"Have you?" the man snapped. He stalked forward, a clear attempt at intimidation. "All I've seen are a few earthquakes."

Jolene considered her response carefully. Here, in the heart of her sanctum, her power was as absolute as it would ever be. She could crush all three men, if she wished. Or kill one of the underlings as an example. Would Bortel react well to naked intimidation? Or was coercion the better way?

She decided on intimidation. It was simple and easily understood. She lacked the time for subtlety.

Jolene raised her hand, the one containing the goblet, and gestured at the armored man on the right, the largest of the three. "Die."

The spell globe at the top of the room, which was tied to a battery of mages whose sole job was fueling its magic, responded instantly to the keyword.

A bolt of negative energy streaked from the globe into the target's chest. Metal, flesh, and bone exploded into particles as the disintegration erased the man from existence.

"Before you draw your sidearm," Jolene began mildly, noting that Bortel's pistol halted halfway out of the holster, as was his remaining companion's. "You should probably know that the globe will respond to me being threatened with instant and terminal force."

"Why?" Bortel snarled, though he didn't venture any closer. "We are allies, damn it. Why kill one of my most capable commanders? How are we supposed to move forward after that?"

"Bortel," she snarled, matching his tone. "You continue to speak to me as if we are equals. *That* is the problem. You assume that we have an agreement. We do not. You work for me, and if that isn't clear, if you think you have your independence, well...I suppose I will have to replace you. There are any number of qualified commanders still left on your world who'd love to be in your position. We've provided ships. The very ships that are about to both save you and make you a very wealthy man. You owe me, Bortel."

Bortel's sidearm snapped back into its holster, and he folded his arms over the armor's chest. "Okay, you've rattled your saber. You've made our relationship clear. Now what?"

The man's professionalism was a wonderful surprise. Perhaps she'd misjudged him. Ah well. He could get another underling. He'd have his pick in a matter of days.

"Nothing has changed. We proceed as planned." Jolene rose from the couch, and approached Bortel, who towered over her. "Over the next seventy-two hours this planet will continue to disintegrate. The very last place to go will be the southern continent, near New Cairo. You set up your little contest, and collect ten legions of the best mercenaries this world has to offer. If you do all that, then I will elevate you to Marshall of my entire army. You will answer only to me, Bortel. I know you hate me, but I can still give you everything you've ever wanted."

"You've got the hatred part right," Bortel agreed. He gave a nod at his remaining companion, who retreated from her sitting room, leaving them alone. "You could have done all this without murder, which shows me that the rumors of your brutality are true. I'll do what you ask, and I'll take that position, but please...no more demonstrations."

"So long as you don't make them necessary." Jolene sipped her wine, and watched as Bortel departed.

She hated that she needed him for what was to come, but if she was to secure a new home world, she'd need the finest troops available to take it. That meant taming Bortel, which she was hoping to do without the theft of will that Nebiat and her blasted Krox had favored.

No, she wanted to break him to her will without the aid of magic. If she failed, well then she'd simply make good on her threat and find a replacement. She had a whole world of mercs to choose from, after all.

Well, for a few more days anyway. Then all this would be a memory.

16

I crept up the last few meters of the ridge, then lowered myself into a crouch next to Rava. She still wore her sunglasses, which whirred as the optics studied the compound below. The rest of her head was covered by a fitted nylon cap that blended with the flurries of snow.

"What do you think?" I whispered, referring to the quartet of guards at the corners of the compound. Two were in crow-nest style towers, while the other two were huddled near doorways leading into the compound, probably so that they could respond quickly to incursions without freezing their appendages off. "Can we sneak past them?"

Rava drummed her fingers along her rifle's stock, and studied the situation. "No. Too much risk."

"She's right," my father whispered as he whirred up behind me on his hoverchair. "Never leave an enemy in your backfield. If your push fails you're caught in a crossfire."

"So how do we get in?" I asked as my father zoomed up next to Rava. I studied them both, looking for some sort of link. Beyond the smile and the eyes there was none.

"We kill them all." Arcan's metal boots crunched as he

methodically plodded up to our position, his lungs working as he moved that much mass at this altitude. He'd left his bald head naked to the snow, and didn't seem to feel the chill. "We have enough shooters to hit all four at once, then we move forward as a group to the ramp."

I nodded, though I still saw some problems. "We're going to need to move quickly. If it were me, as soon as I saw an attack I'd button up, and we don't have the kind of firepower to cut through the hull. They can just sit there laughing at us."

"Good point," my father admitted, which warmed me. His steely eyes were focused on the compound below. The intensity had been absent for so long. "That means we need one person to get inside immediately, without being detected, while the rest of us take down the guards."

"I'll do it," Rava gave immediately.

"No you won't," Arcan countered, frowning at his daughter, his metallic eyes drilling into her. "You're our best sniper. You're on cleanup."

"He's right," I admitted. My shoulders slumped a little when I realized who the best choice was. "I'll go. Briff, you can feint at the first tower, then drop back behind those boulders. While you're doing that, I'll go for the ramp. I can camouflage if needed, and I'll work my way inside when they're focused on you guys."

"You realize," Arcan began, his tone drier than any desert, "that if you screw this up, all of us are dead, right?"

"What the depths is your problem?" my dad snapped as he whirred up to Arcan, and somehow managed intimidating. "Back off. My boy will get it done. He's gotten us this far, and if not for him, you'd be watching your shop float into orbit right about now."

Arcan subsided, though his expression didn't soften.

"I'll get it done," I promised. Having the armor helped with my confidence at least. "Just deal with the guards, and get to that ramp as quick as you can. I will not let them close it."

Nobody looked happy about the situation, and given what we were facing I couldn't blame them. I certainly wasn't happy about it.

I sensed that it was a delicate moment, and it hinged on my next actions. So I crept over the ridge and started down the trail. We'd waited until sunset, and it was close enough that shadows had deepened nicely.

We picked a slow path down, and kept the compound's buildings and the *Remora* between us and where the guards lay. Having a ship in orbit to tell me exactly where they were seemed like an unfair advantage, but their loss, right?

After a tense forty minutes we finally reached the edge of the landing platform where the *Remora* was parked. Briff was bringing up the rear, and while I heard gravel crunch with every step it was more than covered by the wind whistling down from the pass above.

None of the guards had reacted, anyway. If they'd heard Briff I'd expect them to come investigate, but none of the little red dots on my HUD had stirred.

"All right, people," I whispered, just loud enough to be heard over the wind. "Everyone knows what to do. Give me sixty seconds to get into position, then take out those guards. If you hear gunfire before then, engage."

"Got it," my dad growled, his chair bobbing up and down in the wind. He held a serviceable spellpistol cradled in both hands, and I knew he'd be a lethal surprise to anyone who underestimated him simply because he had no legs.

Rava merely nodded, while Arcan didn't even offer that

much. Briff didn't say anything, but I could see I had his full attention from where he huddled under his wings down near a tear in the fence that led onto the platform.

Now or never.

I crept forward, and slowly wormed my way through the hole in the fence. None of the dots moved. I rose to my feet and picked a careful path across the platform, around the *Remora*'s landing struts.

Maybe it was stupid, but I paused briefly and patted the one that had saved my life just a few days earlier. We went way back, that strut and I. Then I crept around the ramp, and my heart rate began to spike.

On the other side of the ramp, twenty meters away, stood one of the guard towers. It was occupied, and if the guard happened to glance down while I was darting up the ramp, if I gave them a reason to turn around....

That would blow the op.

I closed my eyes, just for an instant, and drew on the *fire* in my chest as I channeled an infuse strength spell. Thanks to the armor, I was no longer a weakling. Now, casting the spell made me strong. Really strong, at least by my standards.

One deep breath later I darted from cover, and nearly lost my balance in the snow. If only it could make me graceful. I righted myself, thankful no one had seen.

"Are you even serious?" Rava's amused voice came through the suit's speakers. "Up the ramp, kid. Quick. Like a bunny."

Guess I had been seen.

I scampered up the ramp, wincing at the clatter. None of the red dots inside had moved, though, which meant the first room would be empty. I hurried inside, and took up a position opposite the big red button that would raise the ramp.

I backed the armor up against the wall, and then pulled at the *dream* in my chest. The magic rippled over me, and my armor blended into the wall, invisible to the naked eye. That was the easy part.

Sweat trickled down my brow, and a detached part of my brain considered that a design flaw. I couldn't wipe it away. What if it got in my eyes?

Then one of the red dots began to approach. A moment later a second dot in another part of the ship also began heading this way. That meant that the team had to have killed at least one guard, and that these guys were now aware of it.

I was about to have four lurkers either run past me, or more likely take up firing positions all around me. That's what I'd do, anyway. Set up firing lanes to watch the ramp, and then gun down anyone who came up.

Normally you wouldn't risk leaving the ramp down like that, because your enemy might toss a grenade inside and take you all out at once. Unfortunately, these people had to know why we were here. We wanted the ship, and perforating the hull with superheated metal fragments would render our escape moot pretty quickly.

They held all the cards, and they knew it. Well, they thought they did.

The first lurker charged into view, a heavily cybered merc with a bionic arm and full facial reconstruction. In this case, the enhancements transformed his face into a chrome flaming skull. Cute. He cradled a spellaxe in one hand, each arm thicker than my new legs.

"Roston, get in here! Beck. Stein. NOW!" The beefy merc was clearly in charge, and I wasn't surprised as three more lurkers hustled into view. The leader turned to the last to arrive, an angry-looking woman with a nose ring and a shaved scalp. Also cute. "What's the deal Roston? Who is it?"

"How should I know?" the woman snarled, her voice deeper than I'd expected. She withdrew a spellpistol and took up cover behind a crate.

That shielded her from the ramp, but it put her back no more than two meters from me. Even I couldn't miss that shot.

The last two lurkers both wore environmental suits with helmets, so I couldn't tell which was Beck and which Stein. They flanked the ramp, both cradling conventional assault rifles.

I licked my lips and thought about options. My whole goal had been to prevent them from retracting the ramp, but now I realized that wasn't an issue. The issue was they were going to cut down my friends and family, in a perfect crossfire.

"Here they come!" Roston called, though how she knew wasn't clear. A head implant maybe? Pers-comps were expensive, but maybe someone with money had taken an interest in her.

Well, now or never.

I dropped my camouflage spell, drawing the spellpistol I'd taken from the dreadnought, and sighted on Roston's back. The pistol tore a chunk of *dream* from me, and hit her dead on.

She slumped forward, and elation surged through me.

It evaporated when I realized the other three mercs were turning in my direction.

17

There was one instant of perfect clarity where we all just sort of stared at each other. Then flaming-skull guy started moving, and so did the rest of us. His legs were pumping as he sprinted in my direction, and I did *not* like the look of that spellaxe.

At the same time, both mercs had raised their assault rifles. One had a clear shot, but the other was going to risk hitting their bionic boss. I leaned into that. Literally.

I tumbled forward, taking the merc leader in the legs. There were just two problems. First, the merc was a lot stronger than me, so I just sort of bounced off. Second, there was nothing but my armor to shield me from the merc's automatic fire.

The report told me immediately that I was dealing with explosive rounds.

The first one took me in the shoulder, and something white and urgent and ugly flared there. I was weightless for a moment, then came down in a heap against the wall a couple meters away.

I tried to rise, but my body was being damnably uncooperative. I tried gasping into the comm, but all I managed was a low groan.

"I'm coming, Jer!" My dad's panicked voice came over the comm, from far away.

A shadow loomed above me, and I realized it was the bionic leader, his axe raised in both hands. The muscles in his arms and shoulders all bunched, all working together as he brought that weapon down to end me.

Imminent danger detected, flashed across my HUD. *Full offensive mode engaged.*

Magic rippled from the armor, into me. It was the opposite of the other times. Up until now I'd been powering it, charging it, bonding with it. Now it gave some of that magic back, and did it in a way that would mystify our best artificers.

The axe came down, and my arm shot up. I grabbed the axe blade, and my gauntlet hissed as the glistening green acid coating the blade bit into the living metal.

Power stirred within me, begging for release. I balled my free hand into a fist and aimed it at bionic guy's knee. He laughed. He literally laughed, and just stared down at me.

"You got some moves. You stopped my attack." The merc shook his head in amusement, certain I was about to die. "Go ahead, kid. Take a shot."

"Okay." I shrugged, then I pulled at the *fire* in my chest.

The armor amplified it somehow, feeding it more power, and focusing into a single short pulse that lasted a fraction of a second.

Merc-guy expected me to punch his heavily armored knee from a sitting position where I couldn't bring any of my strength to bear. He did *not* expect me to incinerate his knee, his thigh, and most of the calf.

The suddenly crippled merc spilled backwards with an agonized roar.

I wish I could say that was the end of my problems, but that exposed me to fire from the mercs at the ramp. One of them was laying down suppressive fire to prevent my allies from reaching me, but the other one had calmly aimed his rifle in my direction.

He stroked the trigger, and the rifle bucked back into his shoulder as the explosive round left the muzzle. This was going to hurt.

I managed to get my arms up, but it wasn't enough. The round exploded just outside my faceplate and ricocheted off the wall, black spots blooming as my head rang like a gong. Multiple cracks had spread down the mask, and the paper doll now showed several red spots, and a handful of yellow.

Blinking sent shards of pain through my brain, but the parts of it my father had trained were still working. My trembling fist came up, centered over my assailant's faceplate, and then ejected another pulse of superheated flame.

Everything from the neck up was just...gone. I didn't have time to be horrified as the merc's headless corpse toppled to the deck in a clatter.

The bionic commander had clawed his way closer, and seized my right leg with both his hands. He yanked me back down to the ground, and then heaved himself on top of me.

My infuse strength was still active, and I tried to throw him off, but he batted aside my efforts like a parent disciplining a toddler.

"This is gonna hurt, and I'm gonna enjoy it," he breathed, close to my cracked faceplate, softly, like a lover might. Then he raised his free hand and a pair of razored spurs emerged.

He rammed the blades through my knee, and blood

fountained from the wound. I'd thought the explosive rounds were painful. I was mistaken. Those were merely inconvenient. This was real pain.

It rippled through every neuron, commanding my whole attention. Every part of me screamed one unified message. *Stop the pain, no matter what it takes.*

Both my hands came up, and I wrapped them around the merc's flaming skull. It was hot to the touch, but it was the kind of theatrical heat designed to score points at a bar, not the kind that would hurt me through my armor.

"You like fire?" I snarled, leaning closer and dropping my voice to the same whisper. "This is going to hurt. And I'm going to enjoy it."

I poured every ounce of *fire* I could into the space between my hands, and the armor answered, enhancing that flame. The resulting carnage was sickening, from the smell to the oily residue that burst over my armor and through the cracks in my faceplate onto my cheek.

The flesh boiled away, but the cybernetic skull remained, his electronic eyes staring sightlessly forward as his body went limp on top of me.

I'm not proud of what came next. I had just enough presence of mind to order the helmet to slither off my face, then emptied the contents of my stomach onto the deck next to me.

The dead merc was still pinning me, but that also meant I had cover from his last surviving companion. I craned my head around in time to see my father's hoverchair blur into view.

He dodged a point blank shot from the last merc, which passed cleanly under him. Then my father brought up his pistol in the famous Executioner's Leap that Dag the Slayer had made famous.

He took the lurker in the head, then shot him again in the chest for good measure.

The last lurker clattered to the deck, and I leaned back in exhaustion.

"Yay." I managed a tired little cheer. My infuse strength spell had expired, and I couldn't concentrate well enough to cast another. "Can someone get this guy off me?"

The pain was everywhere, but it was worst in my knee where he'd jammed though spurs. I kept oscillating between passing out and full wakefulness because of the pain.

The pressure on my chest eased, and Rava's face came into focus as she heaved the corpse onto the deck next to me.

"Looks like someone put creamer in their coffee this morning." She nodded at the mess I'd made on the deck. "Guess it was a good thing you didn't have that second helping of eggs."

"Gross." I pulled myself into a sitting position, and rested my back against the wall. "Briff, where are you?"

"Here." The hatchling clomped his way up the ramp. He cradled the railgun in both arms, and the barrel still had steam rising from where snowflakes had landed. "You okay, man? I know humans are supposed to be all pasty, but... you're pretty pale, man."

"Blood loss," my Dad confirmed in a knowing voice. "He'll be fine, if we can get him stabilized and resting."

"We can't do that yet," I protested through gritted teeth. "We need to finish the op. Strip the lurkers, and toss them off the ship."

"What about her?" Rava had picked up the unconscious lurker woman, the one I suspected might have a pers-comp in her head. "She's definitely still breathing. What did you hit her with?"

"Sleep spell," I explained absently, though my mind was on her first question. What did we do? Part of me wanted to lock her up, but doing so meant not only another mouth to feed, but possibly risking the whole op. "I overheard them talking. She's got a link, and I'm betting they can track her. Dump her in the snow with her gear. It isn't much of a chance, but it's more than they gave the *Remora*'s original crew."

My father nodded approvingly, while neither Rava nor her dour father reacted. Arcan had crept in after Briff, but didn't looked like he'd participated in the combat. That didn't much surprise me. If there were casualties, why not let that be your companions so you were in a stronger position?

Having him with us worried me, but that was a problem for later.

"Are you sure, Jerek?" Briff spoke up, though his voice was tentative. "I mean, she's going to die if we leave her behind…"

"If they track this ship," I countered, still through gritted teeth, "then we're all going to die."

"I get it." Briff nodded sadly. The hatchling's tail drooped sullenly, but I didn't budge. Hard choices needed to be made, even if I hated making them.

"What now, Jer?" my dad asked.

"Get to the cockpit and prep for take-off." I closed my eyes and forced several deep breaths through my nose, then continued when the tide of pain abated a little. "If I'm right we've got two prisoners in the brig. I want to interrogate them, and see if they can put some of the pieces together for us."

There was just one problem with my plan. I passed out again.

18

"Jer?" The voice came from a long way away. I wanted to focus on it, but doing so took more effort than usual. My eyes fluttered open, and I became aware of my surroundings.

I'd been moved into an unfamiliar room, and since there was only one room on the *Remora* I hadn't seen, I realized I was in the captain's quarters. Someone had moved me into bed, though I had no idea how long I'd been there or whose bed I was in.

Every part of me ached, but the most insistent pain was still my knee, which throbbed in time with my heartbeat. Something wasn't right there. It felt like my body was hiding the full extent of the injury, somehow.

"Dad?" I croaked, my throat raw and painful.

"Don't sit up." I didn't recognize the emotion in his voice, but it made his words gruff. "Rava dosed you with a stim to get you up. I don't know if it's safe since we don't have a medic. What do you want to do, kid? People are looking for orders, and this is still your op."

I forced myself into a sitting position. The quarters were

dimly lit by running lights in the ceiling, but I could make out the large bed I lay in, and the functional metal night-stand next to it. The walls were bare of artwork, and there wasn't a single decoration anywhere.

"We're still grounded?" I raised a hand to my shoulder, which had also begun throbbing in time with my heartbeat. Everything had a halo around it, which was never a good sign.

"We can take off whenever." My dad whirred a little closer, and I saw the concern etched in normally cynical features. The leathery lines around the eyes were tight. "As long as your wounds don't get infected, I think you're okay, but, Jer...that leg is bad."

"One problem at a time," I countered, trying to give him a confident smile. It hurt. Everything did. "I seem to remember someone teaching me that. Can you have Briff bring me one of the two prisoners? Are we prepped for takeoff?"

"Yeah, we can go whenever. You ready?" My dad whirred over to the doorway.

"Yeah." I forced a nod. Oww. "Get us airborne, and into high orbit. We've got some time before this place comes apart, but not much. I want to know we're safe somewhere, so we can make a real plan."

"Got it." My dad zoomed away. He seemed content to take orders. Happy even.

That got me thinking. My mother had told me about the Peter principle, which had a profound meaning for such a simple name. People get promoted to the level at which they suck. My father had been promoted to a level at which he sucked, but he'd been a god at everything leading up to that. It must be reassuring to be back doing things he knew he was good at.

I wiggled into a better sitting position, which sent a wave of dizziness through me. It abated, but my stomach gave a threatening gurgle promising this wasn't over.

Footsteps sounded in the hallway, then the door pushed open and the pretty lurker I'd first shot with a dream bolt stepped through.

What I'd taken for black or brown hair was in fact a rich auburn, though given that I was shooting at her the last time I'd seen her...and that she'd actually shot me, well, my mistake was understandable. The woman seemed unconcerned by the grease stain on the chest of her overalls.

She was followed by Briff, who really had to work to squeeze in behind her. Had she been a real threat he'd have been completely helpless, but I refrained from pointing it out since the lurker simply stood there staring at me.

Her hair was tied in a simple ponytail, though a few stray threads had escaped. She had clear blue eyes not unlike my mom's, set into a young face. I sensed her apparent youth was deceptive, though. There was a weight to her that suggested she'd seen more than anyone should.

"Your name is Vee?" I croaked, aiming for friendly and landing somewhere closer to noisily expiring.

"Yeah." She folded muscled arms, which didn't at all detract from her femininity, and glanced behind her at Briff, then back at me. "What are you going to do with my brother and me?"

"Your brother," I panted, every word a victory. "He's the other prisoner?"

She nodded.

I didn't even need to think about making such a deal. Leaving that woman behind had cost me, and I was still learning about the price. I wasn't eager to see anyone else die. "If you cooperate and provide actionable intel, then we'll help you get to safety with enough supplies to get you wherever you're going."

"All right." She licked her lips, and moved to sit on the edge of the bed. She barely touched the sheet, an animal ready to bolt if needed. "What do you want to know?"

"Why did the lurkers lock you up?" I rasped, wishing I'd thought to ask Briff to bring me some water. He still lurked by the door, trying to look intimidating, but only managed cramped.

"That's...kind of a long story." She rested her hands in her lap, and darted me an experimental look, as if gauging my mood. "My brother and I are *real* lurkers. That is to say we grew up lurkers. My parents were lurkers. Their parents were lurkers. We never really spent much time on Kemet. I've been shipboard my whole life."

"And the others, the ones upstairs, they weren't real lurkers?" I cleared my throat, and winced as my whole body complained.

"No. About three years ago we showed up at a 'clave, that's a meeting for lurker clans." She raised a hand and stuffed a wayward hair back into her bun. "A new group had showed up. They didn't belong, but they had credits and O_2, and chocolate. Everything we wanted. All they asked was that we tell them when ships were coming up to the fleet from Kemet. Especially ships headed for any of the old dreadnought hulks."

Ships like mine. They'd known we were coming, this confirmed it. And whatever they'd been doing had been going on for a long time. But why? And why now?

I tried tripping Vee up, just in case. Her story was plausible so far, but she'd had plenty of time to perfect it. "After they took over why did these new people keep you alive? They seem pretty ruthless."

"I was born with *life* magic," she explained. Vee raised a calloused palm and it glowed with a soft golden luminance. "It's not strong or anything. But any healing is useful among lurkers. It's how we keep life support running. Anyway, they kept my brother alive as leverage, and because both of us are good with magitech and tech alike. We kept the ships they stole flying, even after...mom and dad."

Despite the surge of empathy it still took everything I had not to beg her to heal me right then, but I knew I needed to keep it together. I couldn't afford to let my guard down.

"Here's the deal I can make you," I promised, though I had to pause before continuing. "If you tend to my wounds, and anyone else who gets hurt, then we will feed you and keep you safe. You'll have to stay in the brig for now, as a precaution. I hope that's acceptable."

"I suppose." She gave a shiver. "I don't like it down there, but I imagine your crew will be taking my old quarters anyway."

I didn't mention that her old quarters had belonged to the people I'd arrived with...before the lurkers had killed them. If it bothered her she certainly didn't show it.

"Are you aware of what's going on down on Kemet?" My breaths were coming fast and shallow, and some sort of morphine was sounding pretty damned attractive.

"You're in pain." She leaned closer, and I saw...compassion? It was genuinely rare enough that I was surprised to see it. She raised one of those rough hands and placed it against my knee. "I can feel it, pulsing. May I?"

I nodded. I wasn't sure I could manage speaking.

Golden light flared around her palm as she pressed it against the sheet over my knee. The magic flowed through her hand, through the armor, and into me.

I'd seen *life* magic used on holo. Everyone had. But very few of us had ever experienced its use. *Life* magic was rare, rare stuff, and only a few thousand mages across Kemet possessed it. There was a reason these people had gone to such lengths to keep this woman alive and working. By contrast there were tens of thousands of void mages, the next most rare.

For an instant I saw divinity. The universe was laid bare, while conscious thought was stripped away. There was no experiencer, only the experience. I became everything, and everything became me. One seamless whole.

Then the light passed, and I found myself blinking. The pain had receded to manageable levels, and none of it came from my leg. As far as my body was concerned, that knee was right as rain.

Vee's eyes fluttered weakly, then she shook her head as if to clear it. "It takes a lot out of me. I can try again later, if you like. Your shoulder must be troubling you."

"I'd appreciate that." I gently pushed back the blanket, and swung my legs over the bed to the floor. I ached something awful, but I was human enough to get back to work. "I'm grateful for what you just did. I'll let Briff take you back to your brother, but I might have some questions later. I'm going to get together with my crew to discuss the situation, and then we'll probably bring you in so we can all have a say."

If I had my way, both Vee and her brother would join our ragtag group. I had a feeling we were all going to need each other in the days ahead.

19

I waited until Briff had disappeared down the ramp into the brig before I headed to the mess and paged everyone through the intercom. That meant that both Vee and her as yet unnamed brother would hear, which is exactly what I wanted.

"All crew, report to the mess, please. We're taking off now, and should be in orbit soon." I released the button, then pressed it again. "We need to get our bearings, people. If there are people you care about, start figuring out where they are."

There was a lot to sort out, and it still wasn't clear what order that should be done in. Vee had added a new wrinkle. If the lurkers were being controlled by someone, and had been for years, then was that somehow connected to the comet? My mom, and through her the prime minister, needed to know that.

I sat down and massaged my shoulder with my free hand. It ached something awful, and I did not deal at all well with pain. Having your world come apart did tend to put minor aches in perspective, though.

"Hey, kid." Rava offered a nonchalant nod as she entered the mess and dropped down at the table opposite me. "You look like the depths just spit you back out, and that's an improvement, sadly. I've been waiting to hear the story. How did you take out that cybernut? He had more chrome than my father and me put together. Not sure I would have come out on top."

I shuddered as my mind drifted back. The aroma of cooked flesh overpowered the present, and I suppressed a gag. I couldn't unsee the exact moment his cybernetic eyes had powered down as the brain that gave them purpose ceased to exist.

"It could have gone either way," I admitted. I looked up to meet her gaze, and found her smiling at me. She seemed like she was waiting for me to continue, so I did. "My armor can use the limbs as thrusters. He thought I was disarmed, because I'd lost my pistol. He was going to finish me slowly, I think. I caught him off guard and...ended it."

It didn't sound terribly heroic, but she gave an approving nod. She kicked both booted feet up on top of the table, and leaned back until the chair creaked. "Not bad. Better than I expected, to be honest. My dad does *not* have a very high opinion of you."

"For good reason," Arcan snarled from the doorway. The dour old man stomped into the room, shoved Rava's feet off the table, then dropped into the discolored plastic seat next to her. "You got lucky, kid, and we all know it." His cyber-eyes whirred as he focused on me, trying to get me to break first.

I knew a power struggle was coming. It would start with logic, and I planned to keep it there rather than escalating.

"Are you sitting inside the ship I promised?" I asked,

quietly, not because I thought it sounded badass, but rather because I was exhausted and couldn't manage much else.

"Yes, yes I am." Arcan delivered a cruel smile, and slowly drew the automatic pistol belted to his thigh, the conventional slug-throwing kind. "Rava, guard the door. The kid and I are going to make a new deal. Play it smart, kid. You can't take me."

Briff had chosen that exact instant to return. The mess had a higher ceiling than the quarters I'd been in, which meant he could stand at his full height, and consequently spent a lot of time here. Never mind that it was where we kept the food.

Rava had drawn her pistol, but was still staring at her father in confusion. That gave me a moment. Just a single moment in which to act. I drew it out, which I hoped would give Briff time to get up to speed.

"You know what, Arcan?" I offered nonchalantly, without rising from the table. I tried to play off the gun in my face, and the exhaustion helped me do that. A small part of me was okay with being shot, because it meant I could go back to sleep. Even if it was the more permanent kind. "You miscalculated on two fronts."

"Oh, really?" Arcan rolled his cyber-eyes. "Why don't you educate me then, kid? Draw from that vast pool of experience you don't have."

"I can't help but notice," I began, making sure I caught Briff's attention. His slitted eyes fixed on me. "...that you don't have a lot of respect for my team's heavy. That's understandable. You've never seen him in action. See, the thing is, if you knew Briff like I do, you'd know that the gun is aimed in the wrong direction."

Arcan snorted a laugh. "Yeah, fatty over there is going to do what, exactly? Rava's got him covered."

That wasn't precisely true. The cybered merc could get her pistol up, but indecision had her in a vice. I could tell she wanted to back her father, but there was a high likelihood she'd hesitate during the critical moment. Especially if I nudged her a little.

"That's the second thing." I tried to imitate Arcan's derisive laugh, but failed. I just sounded like a bad villain in a cheap cartoon. "See, I don't think Rava knows who her real father is. I don't think she realizes I'm her brother. If you're counting on familial ties, well, I've got more in common with her than you do."

It was a huge bomb to drop, one that I wasn't certain was even true. If I was wrong, it was a depths of a gamble, but it was all I could think of in the moment.

It worked.

Rava gaped at me, her pistol held loosely near her waist. "Is—are you—there's no way."

"Ask your 'dad', not me." I nodded at Arcan, and Rava turned that questioning gaze in his direction.

Now.

"Briff," I snapped, with full arena urgency. "Overrun. Now."

Briff is many things. He's slow to deliberate. He's soft-spoken, and not nearly as confident as a dragon should be. But he's got amazing muscle memory.

A dragon's wings are covered by a layer of super-dense scales that make steel look like tin, and if held close to the body act as a second layer of protection. Briff had spent over ten thousand hours playing a game where this was one of his favorite maneuvers.

The hatchling launched himself at Arcan, and even used his tail to push off the deck for additional momentum. Arcan managed to bring his pistol up, and the roar was deafening. The round ricocheted off Briff's scaly wing, leaving it completely unmarred.

Then Briff's much larger, and much, much heavier body crashed into Arcan. The hatchling carried the older man into the wall with bone-crushing force, and pinned him against the steel under his scaly bulk. "You got any more jokes you want to make about my weight, old man? Imma get comfortable, I think."

Briff moved into a better position to crush Arcan into the wall, and Arcan gave an agonized squeak.

Rava started to laugh. It was a cleaner version of Arcan's laugh, with none of the malice. She gasped in lungfuls of air as she pointed down at Arcan, tears streaming from her eyes as his predicament became clear.

"Y-you spend so much time," she wheezed, "talking about how much better you are than anyone. You mocked the kid, maybe my brother, but he came through. You mocked Dag, maybe my real father, which explains a depths of a lot, and he came through. You mocked the hatchling, and hey, look—Briff came through, too."

She wiped a tear away as the laughter finally subsided.

"What do you want me to do with him, Jer?" Briff hauled Arcan up by the scruff of his neck as the merc's feet twitched futilely beneath him

I knelt and retrieved Arcan's gun, which had been lost in the scuffle. I offered it butt first to Rava. "Take him down to the brig, and put him as far from the others as you can."

Rava accepted the pistol, and slipped it into her belt. She folded her arms and gave her father a disappointed look. "You earned this. I'll try to get them to go easy on you, but it's an uphill battle. You know that."

"We aren't going to kill him," I countered immediately.

"He gambled and lost, that's all. We'll hold onto him until we can get things sorted."

"Jer, you're going to want to see this!" My dad came zooming into the room on his hoverchair. He paused in the doorway for a moment when he took in the situation with Briff holding Arcan midair, and a million questions burned in his eyes. Apparently whatever this was trumped it in importance, because he ignored the situation in favor of telling me what he'd found. "You remember War Leader Bortel? Apparently he's gotten himself a full Inuran battle carrier with an empty hold, and is offering to take people off world. The bastard's turning the whole thing into a game. Survival of the fittest. Come on, you need to see this before we make any decisions."

"Then we should all see it." I nodded at the scry-screen on the wall. "Get the broadcast up, but wait for Briff to get back after he throws your buddy Arcan into a cell. Let's see what Bortel is about, and how it impacts us."

20

I t didn't take Briff long to return from the *Remora*'s surprisingly full brig. I waited for him to be seated in the dragon-sized chair installed in the corner, then nodded at my father to play the broadcast. I'd have preferred to view it on my own, but there wasn't time for that. There was never enough time.

Briff sat next to Rava, who elbowed him playfully in the ribs. I caught a whisper, which under other circumstances probably would have made me smile.

"Hey, let's hang later." Rava grinned mischievously up at the hatchling. "Comp stomp! We can blow up some lower ranked teams to get our footing."

My father's chair whirred over the pair like the fabled Sword of Damocles, a legendary Terran deity. Dag scowled down at them, judging them and finding both wanting.

"You scrubs just don't get it," my dad snapped, his rage taking me back a step. I hadn't realized he'd had that much fire in him, but then I realized to whom he was directing it. A daughter whose safety he feared for. "Our world is coming apart. Watch."

He stabbed the button on the holoscreen, and a 3D representation of Kemet sprang up above the device. The world had split through the core, and was slowly breaking into several moon-sized pieces. That wouldn't be apparent to the people on the surface—not yet, other than maybe noticing slightly lighter gravity and some strange weather. Plus the endless quakes of course.

A refined officer's disembodied head appeared on the holo above the world. His face was vaguely familiar, but I didn't place the man until Briff spoke.

"Hey," the hatchling rumbled as he stabbed a claw towards the holo. "That's Bortel. He's in tight with the Inurans. He sponsors more teams than any other war leader, and I hear he just cut some sort of deal for—"

"Shhhhhh," my father interrupted, his glare suppressing whatever Briff had been about to say.

Bortel steepled long fingers, several of which were adorned with enchanted golden rings. Gaudy stuff, but potent. His short dark hair had been slicked back, and shone under the lights. It lent him a dignified air, though to many it would come across as old-fashioned.

"You all know me," Bortel began as he used one hand to stroke a thick black goatee, artfully tinged with grey at the very ends. "I get more and better contracts than any war leader in this sector."

His manner, his clothing, it was all old south, even if our culture had lost the original meaning. Something from ancient terra that signified dignity and hospitality, both qualities mercs wanted to be known for, even if they didn't possess them.

"Now I've got a full Inuran battle carrier," Bortel continued, though he paused dramatically to take a draw from an ornate vape pen before continuing. "It's got an empty hold. Bunks. Chow. What I need are mages. Deadly mages. To that end I've got a proposition. By tomorrow morning most of this planet will be a memory. A day after that there won't be a piece large enough to stand on. You want off? Here's the deal."

The hologram split and the new section showed the Mojave Spaceport, which sat just outside of New Cairo. It was standard fare, and I couldn't see anything particularly alluring about the port beyond sitting all by itself in the middle of a vast field.

"Ladies and gentlemen," Bortel continued in that drawl, "we are going to replenish the legions one last time. I will take a full ten thousand of you. And I know you will be the very best. How do I know that? Because you'll be the ones controlling that spaceport when I land at 7 p.m. standard, tomorrow evening. Survive, and you get to work for me. Or die and be forgotten. The choice is yours."

The transmission ended, and we were left staring at each other. I couldn't believe what I'd just heard.

My hands tightened around the table, and I wished it was Bortel's—or whoever he worked for—neck. "It's certainly convenient that Bortel happens to have a brand new Inuran carrier with an empty hold."

Rava raised an eyebrow and wore her skepticism openly. "You think Bortel somehow arranged for our planet to be destroyed just so he could pick up some mercs on the cheap?"

"No." I leaned back in my chair, struggling to relax. I hadn't put all the pieces together, but I had enough of them that it was starting to make sense. "Someone did, though, and I'm willing to bet that's who Bortel ultimately reports to.

We know that the lurkers were co-opted several years back, if Vee's word is any good."

Briff cleared his throat in an inhuman way that exposed rows of razored fangs. He'd probably meant to be polite, but even a polite dragon commanded attention. "The lurker woman doesn't have any reason to lie. I agree with Jerek. I've been thinking about this a lot."

"Thinking." My dad gave a snort, but he subsided when I glared at him.

"Anyway," Briff continued, now sporting a hurt look. "Jerek knew the planet was going to blow before anyone else. So did whoever the lurkers work for. They're just trying to survive, like we are. Fodder."

"Scaly has a good eye." Rava gave an approving nod as she folded her arms and leaned even further back in her chair. "I don't think the lurker is lying either."

"Assuming she isn't," I jumped in, "then here's what we know. Someone thinks the Vagrant Fleet is important enough to spend billions of credits outfitting lurkers, all so they could keep scavs and relic hunters away. That same someone knew our world was going to get hit, and quite possibly arranged it themselves."

"They're after the old dreadnoughts," my father realized aloud, his jaw falling open. "Bright lady, I see it now."

I waved my hand at the holo, and it shifted to show the Vagrant Fleet, which we weren't all that far away from. Hundreds of hulks floated in a loose orbit, with each mighty dreadnought at the center of its own cloud.

Battle debris still drifted between them millennia after they'd been created. They were trapped by the gravity of the ships, entombed, and one of the worst dangers incoming ships had to deal with.

"The question I'm left asking," I continued, since no

one else had spoken. "What's so important about derelict hulks that it's worth all this? They've been sitting there all this time, but suddenly now they're important? What changed? We need more info, and I can think of a place to get it."

My father's face drained of blood, and his hoverchair whirred back a pace, almost of its own accord. "You're going to call her, aren't you?"

"I am." I nodded, and offered my best encouraging smile. "Dad, you're helping to save what's left of the world. You've got the high ground on this one."

"Maybe." His chair whirred toward the doorway. "Doesn't mean I want to look her in the virtual eye again this soon, especially since she's probably hanging out with my replacement. I'm going to double check the auto-pilot, and see what scans turn up."

Rava rose to her feet as well, then prodded Briff with a booted foot. "If you don't have anything better to do...comp stomp?"

Briff lit up like he hadn't in days, and his wings fluffed behind him as he followed her out of the mess. "What kind of gun do you think I should use? I really like the NTM Cannon. Their stuff is cheap, but its really efficient, and..."

I turned my attention back to the holounit, then adjusted the controls to activate the scry-screen. The holounit was one of the nicest pieces of tech on the *Remora*, and the few pieces of magitech. At some point someone had ripped out the ancient corvette's spelldrive and replaced it with a cheap fusion knockoff, but some other owner had thought to install a state-of-the-art holounit. Thank you, weirdly tech-y person.

That was the way of it with vessels like this. Who knew how old they really were? Some stretched back to planetfall, and judging by the musty smell from this one I wondered. Dozens of diverse owners had likely kept the *Remora* flying.

A bit of *fire* activated the missive, and the scry-screen's edge pulsed red while it waited to connect. The process would probably have been faster had I used Quantum, but listening in on missives was much harder to achieve, and I had a feeling whoever was behind this would be monitoring all communications to the prime minister's ship.

The missive finally connected, and my mother's near-bloodless face filled the monitor. Her composure was back, the professor, but the evidence of her grief remained. She'd been through a lot, and I could only guess at the causes.

"Hey, Mom." I smiled at the holo and took a step closer, almost touching it. "I know you're probably dealing with the evacuation. I just need a minute. You want the good news or the bad news first?"

She gave a tremendously exaggerated roll of her eyes, and then stuck her tongue out at me. Twenty years vanished from her face, and for possibly the first time in her adult life my mother grinned. Not smiled. Not smirked into a hand. She was grinning.

"Are you serious? You *are* the good news. When I heard about the train...well that doesn't matter." Relieved tears flowed down her cheeks as she extended a holographic hand that couldn't really caress my chin. It retracted quickly, and the tears were hastily blinked away. Back to business. "I can't believe you're alive. If there's more good news, let's save it. What's the bad news? It can't be any worse than what we're already contending with."

"You know this attack on Kemet was orchestrated," I began. I wasn't sure how to convey everything I'd learned in an efficient way. "The piece you might be missing has to do with the lurkers. When we retook the *Remora*, this ship, from a band of lurkers, one of the prisoners claimed that there was a power shift a few years back. Lurkers used to be mostly harmless, but then someone with serious funding showed up and started weaponizing them. They've been hitting every vessel that comes near the Vagrant Fleet, including the one I was on. That's why salvage has dried up over the last few years."

My mom cocked her head and adopted a contemplative expression as I spoke, and I had the sense I was filling in a missing piece for her.

"This makes a morbid kind of sense." She glanced off screen, then back. "I'll tell the minister as soon as we're done. She thinks the Inurans are behind the whole thing. Not just the destruction of our world, but also Bortel and his 'contest'. It's not just a way for them to gain legions of mercenaries at a cut-rate price. If our world is destroyed, then our government will answer to those who survive."

That hit me like an asteroid.

"If the Inurans control those legions," I reasoned aloud, "then they effectively control the popular vote for all Kemet citizens. They can control what information those people have access to, and tell them whatever they want."

"And you can bet," my mother added, "that we'll have an Inuran prime minister by the end of the week. What I don't get is what they gain out of all this? What makes this worth all the effort?"

Even as she spoke I remembered my conversation with the dreadnought. A dreadnought more advanced than anything I'd seen or even heard of. More advanced than anything the Inurans could produce today. "The Vagrant Fleet itself. We've been wrong about the hulks for centuries. Our people think of them as salvage, but some of the dread-noughts are still functional. If someone could bring them back online you'd have one of the most powerful fleets in the sector...overnight. They're killing us for our ships."

My mother's horrified expression spoke volumes. "I can't believe even Matriarch Jolene is that monstrous, but I don't see another plausible scenario. We just signed a deal that offered the fleet as collateral if we don't hit a specific financial target when the trade moon arrives. If your lurker intel is right, then this is their endgame, and we're playing catch up while our world comes apart."

I gave a frustrated nod. I hated that we didn't even know who we were fighting.

"I've got a theory I want to investigate in the fleet." I don't know why I didn't tell her everything about my armor, maybe because someone else could be listening. "Are you guys okay for now?"

She nodded, and again glanced offscreen. "I have to go. We're fine, but the minster is trying to find a way to evacuate the academy. They've used their magic to hold that part of the world together, for now at least. All of our greatest cultural artifacts...our libraries. Not to mention the minds who bring all that to life. It's all going to be gone if we can't pull some sort of miracle out of nowhere."

I desperately wanted to cheer her up. I could see her crumbling under an impossible weight, and could only guess what her staff was demanding of her and the prime minister.

"There was more good news." I gave her my best smile, and she blinked expectantly back. "Dad helped get me out, and he's piloting as we speak. Dag the Slayer is...in rare form."

Her eyes shone, though she mastered herself before real tears fell. "That's amazing, sweetie. Your father deserves better than...what I thought you both got. I love you, Jerbear. Stay in contact."

"I will. Love you too, Mom." I reached out to the holo, then killed the connection.

It was time to take the fight to the people who'd been manipulating us, and now I knew right where to hit them.

INTERLUDE IV

Jolene clasped her hands behind her back as she moved to stand at the far end of her office. The entire sitting room had been designed to impress, and the aft wall had been made invisible so the viewer appeared to be dining in space.

It afforded a wonderful view of Kemet's demise, and Jolene had to admit that she enjoyed the world's death struggle quite a lot. Streamers of rocks and debris flowed from many points now, and the planetary fragments were beginning to drift apart. If not for the mages at their precious academy, that part of the world would already be gone.

Fitting, that they should understand what it meant to struggle impotently against much greater powers. Powers as she'd once wielded. Much had been taken from her recently. Her position. Her title. Her divinity, brief as it had been.

In destroying Kemet, Jolene had proven, to herself at least, that she still possessed power. She still mattered. Unfortunately, she'd conducted a good deal of self-examination lately, and had come to a troubling conclusion.

Her mind was eroding, just as Kemet eroded.

Jolene had lost all the trappings of godhood. All the power, the omniscience, and the immortality...gone. She had, however, retained the very worst part of divinity. Hubris.

She was incapable of perceiving the universe as a mortal. Taking into account political niceties now seemed alien. When dealing with Bortel, blunt force had appeared the wiser course. In her mind she was still a god, and therefore her followers should listen. Should know what to do without being told.

That was folly. Today she would rectify that, if such a thing was possible.

Jolene waved a hand, and elsewhere on the ship a fire mage powered the scry-screen. That mage generated a missive, which was sent to Bortel, aboard the very last ship Jolene had been able to procure before she'd fled the Consortium.

The missive connected, and Bortel's ghostly face was superimposed over the invisible wall, the fleet still visible behind him.

"Yes, Matron?" The words were meek, and the man's expression was deferential, yet he couldn't mask his aversion. Not fully.

She considered the merits of an apology, but decided that would only make matters worse. She would address the issue, nothing more.

"How are things proceeding with the contest?" She unclasped her hands from behind her back, and folded them over her chest. The gesture made Bortel flinch.

"Well enough." Bortel stroked his goatee, and struggled to make eye contact. "I suspect we'll end up with eight workable legions, and two trash reserve legions. We've got everything from hovertanks to adult Wyrms jockeying for position. They're already forming their own ranks, which will make our job easier in the long run."

"Excellent." Jolene forced herself to relax, and lowered her arms to her sides. "You've passed every test. I understand you don't know why some are administered, and they may seem like madness, but I assure you all were necessary, and that someday you will understand my actions."

Bortel paused, and looked up then. Naked animosity blazed in those eyes, even if only for an instant. "It isn't necessary that I understand them. I follow orders, matron, and I will do so both swiftly and unerringly until the end of my contract. I can assure you of that."

"I'm sure you will. That will be all, Bortel."

He gave a curt nod, then the missive cut. Bortel was important, in his own way, but not nearly as important as her work in the Vagrant Fleet. It was time to check on that directly. She hadn't risked contacting her people, even with magic, but time was short and she needed answers.

This time Jolene cast her own missive. She raised a hand, and sketched a *fire* sigil in the air, the light blazing as the magic coalesced, heat rolling off the symbol. She added a *dream* sigil, then another *fire*, and then concentrated as the missive completed.

The scry-screen lit, and when it connected it showed the bridge of an unfamiliar vessel behind her chief operative. The walls were forged from a dark alloy that reminded her uneasily of the black ships Talifax had ordered the Inurans to create.

The holo lit and an Inuran man of unremarkable beauty offered a curt nod, though he didn't bother to hide his displeasure at the interruption. "The work will proceed more swiftly without needless oversight."

"I will be brief," she promised, though she hated the meek tone. It ill suited her, but in this instance the expediency outweighed any cost to her pride. "As you haven't reported in, I assume the candidate failed?"

"You assume correctly." Valat's eyes narrowed dangerously. "And before you ask, yes, we recovered the Heka Aten. No, they cannot be used to control other ships. Each is linked to its parent vessel."

Jolene closed her mouth, as he'd just answered her next two questions. She had a third. "How long will it take to train another candidate?"

"It's not that simple." Valat added a frown to the already narrowed eyes, like a feline that had been cornered. "We need a mage who understands both magical theory, and the historical context of the Guardian. In short, they need to think like it thinks. I suspect the reason our last candidate failed was because they were not adequately prepared."

Now it was Jolene's turn to narrow her eyes. She needed this man. For now. "For which you blame me. Very well I will accept that blame. I ordered the attempt before the candidate was ready. We will not make that mistake again. Have you considered entering yourself? You are the most qualified candidate, are you not?"

Greed and fear battled, but the light in his eyes said that fear had won. Valat shook his head. "The risk is too great. If I fail, then there is no one to train additional candidates, and your research stalls."

"I agree with that assessment." And she did. Jolene licked her lips, and forced civility. "Get another candidate up to level 2 in the armor as quickly as possible. This ship is the most important. If we can't bring it online, then none of the others matter."

"I am aware of the stakes." Valat raised a hand to rub his

temple. "I will do all I can. Please do not contact me again. I will let you know when I am ready."

"You have twenty-four hours," she countered, using the sector standard measurement for a single day. "I will contact you tomorrow for a status update, and hope to hear progress. Don't disappoint me, Valat. My patience is not infinite."

Valat paled, all resistance suddenly gone. Apparently word had spread about Bortel's underling. Maybe that had been the right choice after all. "Of course, Matron. I will speak to you then."

21

M y next move was half intuition, but I felt like I was onto something. The ship my armor was connected to, the dreadnought I'd been aboard but whose name I'd yet to learn, was still functional. I knew life support worked in at least part of the ship.

What I didn't know was whether or not the engine, or engines, were functional. My whole plan fell apart if they weren't. It would be damned near impossible to ride to the rescue if the ship wouldn't, well, ride.

There were a lot of problems to solve. A lot of possible roadblocks. A lot of unknowns. But that was the shape of my plan, and I was going to find a way to hammer it into reality.

I'm not attached to much, but every last one of my positive memories growing up came from the academy. I'd fallen in love there, and gotten my heart broken. I'd learned to cast my first spell, and to control the magic living inside me.

More than that the academy was the both the past and future of our people. The past in that it contained the armory, which housed all of the most powerful weapons we'd saved during planetfall. The future in that thousands of cadets in various stages of training called Highspire home.

I'd be damned if I was going to let that all be sucked into the sun.

So I walked my inspired ass down to the brig. I passed Arcan, who glared at me from behind his cell's blue energy barrier. I walked by a curious-looking young man, about my age, with a scruffy beard and frightened eyes.

He strongly resembled Vee, the last cell's occupant. Right down to the shade of auburn in his beard and hair. I moved to his cell, and tapped the red button removing the barrier. I repeated the gesture at Vee's cell.

Both prisoners stared at me as the prospect of freedom dawned, clearly expecting some sort of trick.

"We need to talk," I began, then moved to lean against the wall opposite their cells. "I don't know what life was like among the lurkers, but you've seen holos about the academy, right? You know about Highspire and the armory?"

Vee nodded. Her brother said nothing, and his gaze kept shifting between me and the ramp leading up to the mess.

"I went to school there." I shifted a few steps to the right to block brother's path up the ramp. He flinched, and settled back onto his bench. "I have friends there. Family. And it represents all that remains of three hundred millennia of continuous culture."

"Why are you telling us this?" Vee rose from her bench, and stepped into the hallway, face to face with me. "Are we free to go now?"

"If you help me, then yes." I folded my arms and resisted the urge to draw my sidearm. I was taking an awful chance here, and I knew it. "The dreadnought you originally took this ship on...could you find your way to the bridge?"

"Yes," her brother said, though he didn't leave his bench.

He cowered there, avoiding eye contact. What had they done to this poor guy? "I can lead you there. No need to bring Vee."

"I'll need you both, I think." I drummed my fingers on the suit's forearm, but it did nothing to dispel the nervous energy. "If we can repair the ship's propulsion system, and make sure the life support is stable, then I think we can save about seventeen thousand kids who are about to sucked into the sun, plus what's left of our best weaponry, which I have a feeling we're about to need. What do you guys say?"

"And if we help?" Vee demanded. She folded her arms, mirroring me.

"Then you're full crew," I offered. This was an answer I'd been prepared to deliver. "You both get a full share of all profit, and participate in crew discussions. At the end of the day, though, you accept me as captain. You support my decisions, and agree not to screw over other crew members. Simple enough?"

The pair's gazes met, and something unspoken passed between them. It ended with the man shrugging, then Vee turned her attention back to me.

"I'm in." Vee gave a ghost of a smile, and it lit her face in a way that provoked very unprofessional thoughts. "I thought you were going to ask us to do something dastardly. If you want to get that beast flying, then Kurz and I are your best bet. We grew up making fleet tech work long past its expiration date."

I tried not to seem overeager, but was reasonably certain I came across like a cadet with their hand raised in their very first class. "Do you have any idea what that thing uses for engines? I didn't see anything external, and it would take a lot of power, or magic, to move something that large."

"Gravitic Spelldrive," Kurz said, quietly, and without

raising his eyes from the deck. "We can tell more when we see the bridge, but we'll probably need a mage, or mages, linked to the engines. That's the way all the capital ships were."

"How do you know so much about them?" I asked. We were short on time, but I like to know the people I work with. Plus, it sounded like this guy had access to data I'd never seen back at the academy. No one there could tell us how these things flew, though I didn't tell him that of course.

"Oral tradition," he explained, and finally looked up then. He had clear blue eyes, like his sister's. "Every lurker clan keeps the secrets of their ships, and our religion teaches that each clan originated from their own dreadnought, I mean...if you read between the lines."

"Kurz!" Vee gave a startled gasp, as if Kurz had just revealed something vital. "We do not speak of the maker's accord. He's an outsider."

"He's the captain, and do our traditions not also say to give the captain your allegiance so long as they honor the clan?" Kurz's eyes flashed up from the deck again, this time focused on me. "The old ways are merely remnants of whatever came before. Forgotten procedures that became traditions, and eventually commandments. We don't even remember the name of the god we served, whatever the captains say, yet we still offer him souls."

Vee shook her head, and I sensed this was an old argument. "Traditions form for a reason. We were given a duty, and guidelines to follow to make that possible. It's not necessary that we understand everything. We are not to mingle with the groundbound. We must remain hidden, until the time is right."

"And when is that time, Vee, if not now?" Kurz finally rose from his bench, and I realized he was taller than me, though leaner, with a frame similar to the one I'd had before donning the armor.

Emotions battled across Vee's features, but in the end she nodded up at her brother. "You're right. We will tell the captain what he needs to know, but I will not compromise my faith beyond that."

"Thank you," I said, as I sensed an opportunity to re-enter the conversation. "I don't want you to compromise your faith any more than you have. I just want to save what we can."

"Then we are of similar minds, Captain." Kurz offered a respectful nod, so I returned it.

Vee rubbed her hands together and smiled hopefully at me. "Getting to the bridge won't be easy. That's going to mean a plan. I don't suppose we can eat while we work?"

I blinked a few times, then realized that I'd not thought to offer our prisoners food.

"I'm so sorry. Follow me, and we'll get you something to eat." I started for the ramp, but stopped outside Arcan's cell when I realized he'd stood and was staring at me.

"That's it?" Arcan gave his trademark sneer. "You have a conversation with a couple of lurkers who killed people you worked with, and now they're pals? But I try to exert my very reasonable claim of being the best suited for being in charge, and I have to rot in a cell?"

Damn it. He had a good point, much as I hated to admit it.

"They're not guilty of mutiny," I countered. "That's a huge difference, Arcan. I know these people are ruthless, but they have skills I need, and they haven't betrayed me yet. You have. And you and I both know you will again."

"You can't keep me in here forever." His cyber-eyes

whirred menacingly as the irises narrowed to little red dots. "I will find a way out."

"Out the airlock, if you keep this up." I turned from Arcan without another word and headed up the ramp.

"What's the story with that guy?" Vee asked as she jerked at thumb in his direction.

"He's a real charmer. Arcan helped us get off Kemet, and we owe him for that." I glanced down one last time as the brig vanished from sight. "He's right that I can't keep him in there, but he's the very last person I want behind me with a gun."

"He'll be trouble," Kurz offered quietly. His gaze had fallen to the deck again, though it was clear he was listening intently to everything around him. "It would be easier if you spaced him. Or suffocated him and salvaged the cyberware."

"You have no idea how tempting that sounds," I confirmed as we entered the mess and headed for the table in the far corner. "Unfortunately I think we're going to need him for my plan to work."

22

By the time I had assembled the crew in the mess, both Vee and Kurz had finished gorging themselves on the vanilla protein paste we'd found in the ship's larder. They sat waiting, Vee with a spot of vanilla paste on one cheek. She glared at my friends confrontationally while Kurz kept his eyes glued to the deck.

How was I going to get these people to work together?

"So here's the plan," I began, my tone as confident as one semester of public speaking could make it. "We are going to land on a dreadnought surrounded by dense debris, sneak past lurker guards, and make it to the bridge. Once there, Vee and Kurz are going to repair the engines. Then we'll pilot the ship back to Kemet to rescue the academy, and arrive as big damned heroes of old. I know you've got questions. Let's deal with that, then Dag will pilot us through this mess."

The plan sounded ludicrous to me, with failure points everywhere. But they watched me expectantly. All of them.

"What about my dad?" Rava asked, her jovial manner smothered by the question, and the answer she probably feared. Her leather jacket creaked as she leaned forward in her chair. "Is he involved in this plan? And, uh, if not, what are you going to do with him?"

"That's one of my very first questions." I moved to the holo, and called up an image of the dreadnought we were making for. "When we land we're going to have to make our way from the aft cargo hold all the way to the bridge. Like all early capital ships, the corridors are wide enough for small vehicles..."

"...And we just happen to have a rover," Rava finished for me. Her confident grin was back. "You need my dad to drive the rover and get us to the bridge."

"We do." I nodded. "In exchange, we forgive him for his misguided mutiny."

"Oh, come on." My dad whirred a little closer, and stabbed an accusing finger in my direction. "Arcan is absolutely, one hundred percent going to screw us over the first chance he gets."

"No, he won't." I folded my arms and met my dad stare for stare. It wasn't easy, but I knew I was in the right. "We need him, Dag. Arcan will screw us, but not until it aligns with his interests. If we succeed, and take the dreadnought, then he gets a full share of the loot, alongside the rest of the crew. If he screws us over, he dies too."

My dad growled low in his throat. "You don't get it, Jer. We can't trust him."

"Which is why," I countered as I raised a hand to forestall his protest, "*you* are going to watch him. When we make our run to the bridge, you ride in the cockpit, and keep Arcan company. Arcan won't need a sidearm to drive, and I'm sure he'll understand that you're only there for his safety."

My father adopted a predatory grin. "I stand corrected. Good plan, son. I'll keep an eye on that snake."

"Any other questions?" I turned my attention to the rest of the crew. Rava and Briff were whispering in low tones, and seemed to have missed the entire exchange.

Vee was watching, and Kurz listening, but neither said anything.

"All right, let's do this. Dag, take us out. Vee, will you handle navigation? Or have your brother do it if he's more qualified?" Issuing the orders was getting easier, and to my surprise both Vee and my father started up the narrow corridor toward the bridge.

The *Remora*'s bridge was designed for up to four people, each sitting at a nearly identical terminal. The deck sloped downward into what would be the head of the creature the ship was named for, and the lower tier of stations faced a wide, curved holoscreen that currently displayed the space outside the ship.

Cramped, but functional. And did I mention ancient?

My dad moved for one of those terminals, while Vee slid into the other. I dropped into the back row, and watched as my dad expertly guided the craft through pre-flight.

"You've flown a lot?" Vee asked as she studied him from the navigator's station.

"Yup." My dad settled his hands around the manual controls, which were totally alien to me. A spell matrix I could use, but a joystick? Not so much. My dad cleared his throat. "I used to be pretty good, but truth is I'm rusty. Haven't navigated this part of the fleet since before you were born."

The ship rumbled as the *Remora*'s drive engaged, and we moved smoothly toward the debris field in the distance. My father used a feather touch on the controls, which I'd seen

many times over my lifetime. He'd flown Mom to confer-
ences, and had taken me to more than one tourney he'd
been competing in.

Age hadn't dulled his abilities, and we zoomed around a
cracked thruster as he took us into the debris field. We
moved slowly, and my dad feathered the thrusters to control
the drift. We began to corkscrew at an odd angle, and the
fleet spun drunkenly on the monitor.

To anyone watching we were just one more piece of
debris that happened to be floating toward a dreadnought's
gravity well.

The holoscreen adjusted for the spin before I lost my
lunch, and I watched as my dad guided us around the first
derelict vessel, a corvette class that had been stripped right
down to the registration.

"This is the first observation point," Vee whispered. She
reached for her terminal, and the lights dimmed all over the
ship. "I am minimizing our heat signature, though if they
are watching, odds are good they already spotted our
passage."

"How can we tell?" I asked. My hands tightened on the
console before me, though I was careful not to touch the
controls, as they were unfamiliar.

Vee spun her chair in my direction, her voice a bare
whisper. "We cannot. However, if they did see us they may
not wish to risk a signal, as they know we will be listening. If
they're lazy they'll wait to see if we make it back out, then
pounce on us to take our salvage and the ship."

Hearing such a beautiful woman so callously relate
murder and piracy rocked me to the core. I liked Vee, but it
was important to remember that we came from different
worlds, with very different moral codes. Azure drakes were

pretty, but that didn't mean you wanted to be in a jungle with one.

"Quiet," Dag whispered over his shoulder. "Trying to concentrate."

I glanced at the holoscreen, and my father had guided us past another vessel, this one a frigate, also picked clean. The debris was getting thicker, and it was taking more micro-adjustments to ensure we didn't hit anything.

Something clanged off the hull like the sector's largest gong being rung, and I winced, then turned to my terminal to see if I could run some sort of damage diagnostics.

I'm not terrible with computers, just inexperienced, and most operating systems are fairly friendly if you're patient and read the help screens.

"Looks like we're okay," I said, as soon as a schematic of the ship appeared on my console. "Superficial damage to the hull, but beyond scoring the paint I think we're fine."

"Keep those scans internal," Vee hissed. She shot me a look that said I should have known better.

I nodded, and shut down the scanner. I didn't like being reminded that I wasn't exactly qualified to be leading this. I was the best we had, though. I firmly believed that. If I really thought someone like Arcan could have guided us through safely I'd have turned over control.

But he wouldn't. So I couldn't.

"There she is," Vee breathed as she pointed at the holo.

I leaned closer and got my first real look at the dreadnought where the armor had come from. Sure, I'd seen it last time we approached, but back then it had just been a scary old hulk. Now it was a potential lifeline.

"We aren't the first ones here," Dag whispered. He nodded up at the holo, his voice hoarse. "That's an Inuran frigate bolted to the hull right over the bridge. She'll only hold about twenty-five people, but you can bet all of 'em will be battle-hardened mages in state-of-the-art gear. Expect spellarmor and potions. If they're all near our target...we might as well turn around."

I shook my head emphatically.

"And go where? We're committed. Besides, we have a plan. It will be all right." I mean, I knew it wouldn't, but I still hoped I could allay my dad's fears. "If the plan works, then my magic will keep them from detecting our approach. We'll get the jump on their position with the benefit of full armor. Even spellrifles aren't going to puncture that rover, whereas our turret will wreck even the best Inuran spellarmor if they get hit. And I've got the Heka Aten armor. We'll be able to track the Inurans' movement. We'll know where they are, and be able to avoid them."

My father shook his head. "It's flimsy and I still don't like it. There are a lot of if's in this plan, and I can tell you all about how that turns out."

"You have until we land to think of a better option." I rose and turned from the cockpit. "I'll get everyone into the rover. Get us docked, then get down there. We're doing this."

23

My hand shot up and seized one of the rover's cargo rings as the entire ship lurched. Briff tumbled into the rover's wall with a grunt, while Rava simply stood there like a Terran sailor weathering a storm.

Vee and Kurz were both seated and buckled in, probably because they'd expected the rough landing.

Arcan barked a bitter laugh from the driver's seat, which was separated from the cargo compartment by a thick metal grate. The holes were small enough to stop a projectile, though they wouldn't do anything to stop a spell unless they'd been enchanted, which I doubted.

"Get the engine fired up, Arcan." I gave the order knowing he'd been about to do it anyway. That had been one of the first leadership lessons my dad had taught me as a kid. Give basic orders that people were going to do anyway, and they'd get used to following you.

Somehow I didn't think Arcan would be that easy.

"Done." Arcan flipped several switches on the dash, and

the rover's power plant rumbled to life. The high-pitched whine it emitted would carry, but theoretically that was where I came in. Arcan turned back to face me, those scarlet cyber-eyes somehow conveying his judgement. "Change of plan, 'Captain'. I don't need a babysitter. We're going now."

Arcan turned back and the rover lurched into motion. We were across the cargo hold, and halfway down the ramp before I could even formulate a response.

My hand slid down to my sidearm, and I drew the black pistol I'd taken from the dreadnought. I pressed the barrel against a hole in the grate right behind Arcan's head. My voice was much calmer than I thought I'd be able to manage. "Are you sure you want to do this, Arcan? I'm not big on third chances."

"Trust me." The rover rolled to a halt inside a cavernous cargo bay, maybe the very same one I'd landed in the last time. If it wasn't, then it was close to identical, which made sense. Arcan flipped another switch, this time activating an audio connection with the *Remora*. "Dag, we're changing the plan. We're going without you. Keep the engines hot. We might have to fall back in a hurry."

"Yeah, no," my father's snarkiest voice came back through the speakers. "There's no way I'm trusting you with...my son. Turn that thing around. Right now, Arcan."

"Dad," I called, letting him know I was listening, "do you think Arcan is right about keeping the ship hot as a fallback point?" The barrel of my weapon hadn't wavered, and Arcan had to be aware of that.

"Yeah, probably." My dad hesitated. "It doesn't change the fact that we can't trust him."

"Rava," I called, drawing her attention away from the conversation she'd been having with Briff. "Take the turret.

Dad, keep the ship hot. Vee, I want you up front covering Arcan. If you suspect him of betraying us, shoot him."

I removed my pistol and offered it to Vee. She nodded as she accepted the weapon, then slid the rover's door open and moved to the passenger's seat next to Arcan. Kurz watched her go, but said nothing.

My dad was silent for a long time, and I winced when he finally spoke. It was much better than I'd expected. "Orders received. Good luck in there, team. I'll keep our ride ready."

I settled back into my seat, satisfied with how I'd handled that. "Let's get moving, Arcan."

Arcan gave an amused snort. "At least you can see reason. Just keep us quiet, and I'll get us there."

This next part relied exclusively on me, but was pretty simple when you got right down to it. The camouflage spell I was always using doesn't have to work on sight. You can choose any sense...which includes sound.

I closed my eyes and rested my hands on the metal wall next to me. *Dream* bubbled up from my chest, then flowed into the armor, and finally into the rover. I grunted from the strain, as covering something as large as a rover was much more difficult than blending myself into a wall.

No visible change occurred, and the people inside could still speak as normal. Anyone outside would hear nothing suspicious. Any sounds we made would be transmuted into sounds you'd expect from a hulk of this age.

Sustaining the spell would take effort, but not concentration. I'd be free to move on to the next phase.

"We're good," I managed through gritted teeth.

Arcan turned on the headlamps, and rolled up the first corridor. I closed my eyes again, and willed the helmet to slither over my face. Once the HUD lit, I sat down and got to work.

"Okay, dreadnought," I muttered aloud. "Why don't we start with names? I'm aboard, so the interference should be gone. Feel free to introduce yourself."

"As you wish." A translucent grey-scaled hatchling appeared in my vision, a holographic overlay provided by the armor. The hatchling wore armor similar to mine, and carried an ornate dragon-headed staff with a thick silver haft in one hand. "You may call me Guardian. The vessel you are aboard is designated the *Word of Xal*."

I gaped at Guardian. This was so far beyond what I'd expected, but it changed nothing. I had a job to do.

"Okay, Guardian," I said, more confidently this time. "I need you to provide an overlay of the area around the bridge. Plot our approach, and take us along the safest route. Our objective is to avoid attention. I want a scan of all lifeforms in the vicinity, and those should be displayed as red dots."

I shook my head in disbelief. I hadn't even finished speaking, and as I uttered each order my overlay shifted to provide the requested data. I could see a cutaway of the bridge and the levels around it, including our route in, which was marked in blue.

Our destination was marked in gold, and a timer said it would take about six minutes to reach it. That was helpful.

Several red dots appeared on the bridge, and a half dozen appeared in a cluster just outside of it. The rest were divided into groups of three, and appeared to be patrolling parts of the ship.

There were also four static locations where trios of stationary dots waited. Each was a major strategic choke-point, and we were going to have to pass right by one of them.

"In two minutes," I said into the comm, "we're going to

reach a T-intersection. I'm marking your maps to show where the defenders are. They shouldn't hear our approach, but if they react in any way I'll notify you immediately."

We rolled along in silence, the tension so thick we didn't need words. I knew, based on my map, that we were approaching the first group of soldiers at full speed. And that they were likely hiding behind some sort of portable barricade. Even bargain mercs have access to that kind of tech. The Inurans would have much better.

I was about to ask Arcan about it when the rover abruptly sped up. I glanced through the grate, through the dash, and up the darkened corridor in time to see our head-lamps illuminate the Inuran position.

I'd seen enough holos to recognize a professional setup when I saw one. A two-meter barricade blocked the corri-dor, and the defenders were huddled behind murder holes so they could fire back at us.

A barrage of white and blue spells shot from the barri-cade, and the hair rose on the back of my neck as they slammed into the rover. Fortunately, the armor was thick and the Inurans were primarily using light bolts. Lasers, basically, for the non-magical folk.

Arcan floored it. The rover hit the barricade going 180 KPH, far faster than I'd have imagined the rover capable of without a longer straightaway to build up speed.

The barricade was forged from some sort of lightweight alloy, which made sense. Otherwise they'd never be able to move it around and set it up. Unfortunately, that constrained them to the laws of physics. Magic could strengthen metal, but only to a point.

Our rover weighed a good four or five thousand kilos. When we slammed into the barricade it ripped loose from the floor, and slid backwards with a tortured shriek and a

shower of sparks. The defenders were completely unprepared, and tumbled to the ground as their own barricade
scooped them like a plow.

Then both rover and barricade met the opposite wall,
and I was suddenly weightless.

24

F or one terrifying moment the rover sailed through the air as it ricocheted off the far wall. Had the ceiling been higher, or the walls wider, then we'd have absolutely flipped. Instead the corridor constrained our movements, and all that kinetic energy was channeled into us rolling backwards.

"Targets acquired," came from behind me, and I glanced back to see Rava inside the turret's control console. "We've got four hostiles still moving. Warming up the cannon."

That was my cue.

"Lay down suppressive fire," I roared, imitating my dad. "Keep them under cover until that turret can fire." I reached for my pistol before realizing I'd loaned it to Vee.

No problem.

I raised one of the suit's armored fists to the slit in the rover's side, right around eye level, and then I reached for the *fire* in my chest. The gauntlet ejected a bolt of super-heated flame, which caught an Inuran mage in white spell-armor just as he rose to his feet.

The bolt hit him in the thigh, but the armor deflected

the spell. He gave a grunt of pain, then aimed a spellrifle at the rover. A bolt of electricity crackled from the barrel, then grounded into the rover's frame. That much ferrous armor bled off the energy, insulating us from the brunt of it.

Automatic pistol rounds came from Arcan, who'd pinned another mage behind a twisted hunk of barricade. Behind me Briff gave a frustrated curse, and I understood why. He couldn't fire his spellcannon unless he went outside, and there was no reason to leave a protected position.

Vee and Kurz merely watched the situation play out. Neither used a spell, or contributed in any way. I considered saying something, but given that we were winning I wasn't sure what that would be. Hopefully they'd be more active when we actually needed them.

Had I been wrong to trust them? I was starting to worry.

No time.

I loosed another fire bolt, and this time I caught my target in the faceplate. The spell knocked him into the wall, and I followed up with another.

An unexpected opponent shot to its feet, this one wearing heavy spellarmor and carrying a spellshield. They stepped in front of my target, and the spellshield came up smoothly to block my spell. The flame rippled harmlessly off the glowing blue runes on the shield's surface, and the figure raised a spellcannon to return fire.

The barrel glowed with a deep violet light, and a bolt that hurt my vision flashed toward the rover. It impacted over Vee's head in the passenger compartment, and everything it touched simply ceased to exist.

"Disintegration!" Arcan roared from the driver's side.

"Any time, Rava," I shrieked, and yes, it was a shriek. A manly shriek.

The whine from the turret grew in intensity, then something beyond hearing pulsed through the corridor. Vee and Kurz both clutched their heads, though my armor protected me from the worst of it.

The entire rover slid back three meters as the gauss rifle discharged a hunk of brittle metal at supersonic speed. To their credit the mage got their spellshield up in time to block, but the shield wasn't designed to stop a round that could puncture ship hulls.

The kinetic force slammed the mage into the wall, and what was left didn't so much as twitch, much less try to rise.

That exposed my target, and I loosed another fire bolt. It caught the mage in the knee, and they stumbled into Arcan's pistol fire. That one went down too, and I was shocked to realize that was the last one.

"I think we just won," I muttered into the comm. "Status report. Sound off."

"Green," Briff gave immediately, following the accepted arena custom.

"Green," Rava panted, out of breath for some reason. She grinned at me from the turret. "Did you see what I did to that guy?"

"Green," Arcan growled from the front seat. "Kid, we need to get that barricade out of our way. They know we're here now."

Neither Vee nor Kurz responded to the sound off, and I didn't have time to teach them. Arcan was right.

"Briff, let's get that debris moved. Rava, cover us with that turret." I popped open the side door and hopped out, then hurried over to the mangled barricade.

I tried to ignore the stench of blood and ozone, and tried even harder not to stare at the severed hand still clutching a sleek white pistol.

Instead I focused on lifting the barricade out of the path of the rover, which was considerably easier than I'd expected, both because of my newfound strength, and because Briff was doing most of the heavy lifting.

We heaved the barricade out of the way, then rushed back into the vehicle's cargo compartment.

"Captain," Kurz said from his bench, without looking up at me. "I know time is precious, but may I exit the vehicle, just for a moment? I wish to claim this man's soul. If I do not do so it will be lost. He was a worthy adversary, and I would honor him. If it matters...this will also fuel my magic, and increase my effectiveness against our enemies."

"Make it quick," I ordered, almost without thinking. Kurz leapt into action, and Vee followed.

Since we were stopped anyway, I followed the pair to see exactly what Kurz meant by claim a soul.

"Kid," Arcan called from the driver's side window as I passed. "We ain't got time for this. Seconds count."

"I realize that." My gaze never left Kurz, though I stopped next to Arcan's window. "We're going to be racing those other teams back. Here's the thing. If we engage now, and they come up behind us, then we're surrounded. No pulling back. If we wait a little longer, and they've all pulled back...well, at least all our enemies are all on one side."

"Yeah," Arcan snapped, his eyes whirring into a menacing expression. "The side we are trying to get to. This is a mistake kid."

"Maybe," I allowed.

Kurz had knelt next to the severed hand, all that remained of the mage I'd killed. He withdrew an ornate crystal vial, what my professors would have called a phylactery, and gently opened the stopper with one thumb.

He brought his other hand around, and sketched a trio

of sigils in the air. I recognized all three, even if I couldn't use them. Sickly white *spirit*, then clear azure *water*, then *spirit* again.

A sort of...cloud rose from the hand, and coalesced into a spectral version of the armored figure. She removed her helmet, and long dark hair spilled out. Kurz waved his hand, and the cloud flowed into the bottle, as if being suctioned.

Once the flow had stopped, Kurz stoppered the vial and slipped it into his pack. He gave me a brief nod. "We can go. Apologies for the delay, Captain."

I had so many questions and no time to ask them. By the time we hurried back into the rover Arcan had begun snarling wordlessly under his breath.

"Okay, let's go. Now." I slammed the door, then buckled myself in. "Arcan, any suggestions on our approach? Should we change it up since they know we're here?"

"Naw," he growled as we whipped around another corner, and started up a gentle slope toward the bridge. "Our only advantage is speed. We get there and assault them as hard as we can go, and hope we overwhelm them before they can pull back the teams from the rest of the ship. This is our one shot, and that window will close quickly."

I considered that for a moment, then tapped the grate behind his head. "Okay, let's do it. Get ready, people. This next part is going to be harder."

The rover whipped down the corridor as we approached the next group of dots. I took a few moments to study them, as well as the movements of the other dots. "They've started collapsing back to the main ship, but they're still moving. We'll get there after them, but just barely, so they won't have much time to set up."

"They're already set up," Arcan roared as he darted a

glare over his shoulder. "By the time we arrive they'll have heavy weapons online. This is going to be messy. Hold on."

A sharp whistling filled the vehicle as the air rushed through the missing section of the roof, loud enough that it would have overpowered any conversation...had there been any. We were all worried, and with good cause.

As leader I knew I should offer a rousing speech, but I had nothing to give. No idea what to expect, and no way of knowing if this was the right choice or suicide.

My hands tightened around the cargo ring as we raced closer. I'd used some of my *dream* to camouflage us, and some of my *fire* in the last fight, but I should be good for another round.

"Get ready!" I called as we entered the final approach.

As before, Arcan floored it, and the rover picked up speed. The walls flashed by, faster and faster. Arcan killed the headlamps, and suddenly we were hurling through darkness.

There was a soft white glow at the end of the corridor, but I could see neither enemy troops nor a barricade as before. I wondered why, then we burst from the corridor into a maintenance bay and the answer became clear.

The Inurans had used gravity magic to affix their weapons to the ceiling. Four tank-busters, a well known conventional missile, were aimed in our direction. The dots were all still in the room, but they were attached to the ceiling as well, either through magboots or magic.

The concentrated fire they unleashed was beyond impressive. A rain of certain death converged on our position, and the universe exploded into flame and pain.

25

Т he restraints yanked me first in one direction, then another. Had I not been wearing armor I didn't want to know what it would have done to my body. We came down with a thunderous crash, then the vehicle flipped several more times until we came to rest against a wall.

The armor protected me through it all, but as I got my bearings I realized not everyone had the benefit of armor. Arcan was unconscious in the driver's seat, and the dash had caved in, trapping his legs. There was blood everywhere, though I could see the vein in his neck throbbing, which I took as a good sign.

The passenger compartment had ceased to exist, and the ceiling in the cargo compartment was a good meter shorter than it had been. I heard groans from all around me, another good sign.

My latch wouldn't unhook, so I used a bit of *fire* through the gauntlet to burn through the belt itself. "Sound off. Who's still conscious?"

"Oww," Briff rumbled. "One of my wings isn't working, but I can still fight. Cannon checks out. Green."

"Green," Rava called next, though I noted the quaver in her voice. I glanced at the turret console, which had weathered the explosion mostly intact. She had blood streaming down one arm, but seemed otherwise unharmed.

"Kurz is unconscious," Vee called. There was a tightness to her voice I recognized. Pain.

I twisted in what remained of my seat to get a look at her. She was the closest to the door, which had been warped out of the frame. That left about a half-meter gap for us to crawl through.

"They're going to be covering our exit." I wiggled closer, next to Vee, until I had a view through the gap. "Can you see anything?"

"Two of the missile emplacements," she said, her face near the gap, but not close enough to present a target for a sniper. "They're both empty."

"T-they fired all four," Arcan rasped. He coughed, then shook his head as if clearing it. "Amazed we survived that. Guess the enchanted frame was worth it, or we'd be nothing but a smudge. Looks like I'm a permanent part of the rover now, though."

"Dad?" Rava crawled from the turret, over to the grate. "Did it hit an artery? If not, I can cut you free in a couple minutes."

"We don't have minutes." Arcan's cyber-eyes whirred. He raised a quavering hand and placed it on her shoulder. "You turned out all right, kid. Your mother would be so proud."

Rava began to tear up, the first crack in her exterior I'd yet seen. Arcan gave a bitter laugh, and the tears vanished. He turned his cyber-eyes in my direction. "You got a plan, Captain? I'm stationary, but I'm still an asset."

I glanced at the gap in the door again, then back at my team. My team. "Vee, you've got *life* magic. Can you manifest some sort of ward?"

She nodded, and when she spoke her voice was a bare whisper. "I can erect a powerful ward. It will not last long, but it should stop spells and projectiles for a short time."

"A very short time," I corrected. "If it were me I'd counterspell the ward the instant I saw it. Rava, can that turret still fire?"

"I don't know." She turned from her father, her determination returning now that she had a task. She began squirming toward the turret.

"It will fire," Arcan said. His teeth were gritted now. The pain must be unreal. "And I can control it manually. It's got a limited field of motion, but I can hit the ceiling with it."

I considered our assets. A bad plan was better than no plan. "Here's how we'll play this. Vee, I want you to cast your ward. Expect it to get popped immediately, and be ready with another. Keep casting wards until I say go. We're going to bait them out. When we're ready to actually move, Arcan will fire the turret at their position. We apply another ward, then bolt from cover. Vee, can you move with that ward?"

"No, but if you carry me I should be able to maintain it."

"Briff, your spellcannon will be important at the break." I stared down at Kurz. "Rava you're going to be hauling Kurz to safety. Briff you keep the suppressive fire going, and we beeline for the corridor we came in through. Not great, but it's what we got. Any feedback before we do this?"

Everyone shook their head.

"Guardian, update my display to show all current enemy positions, including weaponry." A moment later my HUD updated, and several grey dots were added to represent the hopefully empty missile batteries. "I don't suppose you can assault these guys with some sort of internal defenses?"

"Negative," Guardian's voice came from my left, and I shifted to see his holographic form on my HUD. "Only a full captain may unlock the weapons systems."

Well, it was worth a try.

"All right, people. We begin when Vee erects the first ward." I leaned back against the wall. In a minute I'd probably be running. May as well enjoy being lazy for a minute longer.

Vee extended a shaking hand, and a silver bracelet around her wrist flared with an inner brilliance. I'd never seen it before now, which shocked me. I'd definitely have noticed that. As would her previous captors. How had she hidden the artifact?

A shimmering ward sprang forth, whirling outward in concentric rings as it formed a dome over the gap in the door.

The ward hadn't even finished forming when a volley of spells converged on it. A counterspell may have been among them, but it hardly mattered. The ward shattered after a few moments of abuse.

She cast another, with the same result. And another. And another. On the fifth I noticed a trickle of sweat. She paused before the sixth, and faced us. A single auburn hair wove a line down her face, but she ignored it. "I cannot do many more. Are we ready?"

"Ready," Arcan managed, though it triggered another cough. "I'll fire on three?"

"Do it." Only in that moment did I realize that Arcan was signing his own death warrant. These people didn't seem interested in prisoners. "My dad was wrong about you. Thank you, Arcan."

Rava sobbed behind me. I thought about offering comfort, but realized she'd hate that. I focused on the fight, and brought her into it. "Rava, get Kurz up. Briff, get into position. We're doing this when Arcan hits three."

"One," Arcan roared, his voice clotted with pain. "Two. Three!"

Briff burst from the vehicle with a tremendous kick that sent the door flying. Several marksmen shot the door on instinct, which was a few more not firing at us.

Vee came next, and quickly erected another white dome, the shimmering ward expanding to three meters, just enough to cover our position.

The gauss cannon fired, and a hunk of metal slammed into a cluster of Inuran mages on the far side of the roof. They tumbled to the ground like distant bugs, though all were still moving.

I rolled out, then turned to help Rava with Kurz. She hit the ground and slung him in a fireman's carry, just as volleys of spells hit Vee's ward. It shimmered, but held.

"I can't do this long!" she yelled, her voice at panic's edge.

"Go!" I sprinted toward the opposite door, and the rest followed.

Briff fell instinctively into the rear, and his good wing came up to shield us as the ward went down. He roared in pain as several spells slammed into the leathery section in the middle, and I watched in horror as a wide swath of scales was disintegrated.

Vee cast another ward, which intercepted the final volley as we made it into the tunnel. We'd gotten incredibly lucky in that the vehicle had landed near the corridor. Had we been at the opposite side, our deaths would have been a casual matter for the Inurans.

Her ward dropped, but we were up the corridor and out of their line of fire. Thanks to the armor, sprinting was easy, and everyone else seemed to be managing.

I moved immediately to Briff, who was still limping at the rear. Both wings hung behind him, tattered and broken.

"Hey, Jer." Briff panted as he trotted, and I fell into step behind him.

"How you holding up, bud?"

"I look that bad?" Briff offered a toothy smile, which reassured me. He hadn't lost his humor.

"Not that bad," I lied, then glanced back behind me to avoid eye contact. There was nothing to celebrate, other than survival.

Arcan wouldn't be so lucky.

INTERLUDE V

Inura's tail thrashed in agitation as he gazed at the intensely intricate spell dominating the containment chamber where he was testing the latest iteration of his schema. There were inefficiencies that must be eliminated before he could go any further, yet he'd been at this ninety hours without a break.

It was time for clarity.

He strode from the workshop and stretched his wings. The motion relieved tension, and he rolled his shoulders to loosen his arms.

Inura's body had many advantages. It appeared human, if one overlooked the slitted irises, tail, and wings. Closer examination revealed that the pores of his skin were really scales, a much better defense.

He appeared just mortal enough that mortals didn't flee in gibbering terror, as they would if he appeared in his full Wyrm body. Well, the Wyrm body he'd used to possess.

Like it or not, and he most certainly did not like it, this was his only body now and the sum of his power. Everything he'd been, all the power and magic he'd amassed in his ancient draconic form, belonged to the *void* now.

That had been the price of his survival.

He had infused a simulacra, what his sister had called a shade, with half his power and all of his memory. That had proven prudent. He'd scryed the battle, and seen himself die. It was...unsettling, to say the least.

Inura continued up the corridor into his spacious chambers, which were littered with books and knowledge scales. He'd never been very tidy, and becoming a god hadn't changed that.

He considered picking one of them up to relieve the tension and boredom, but nothing interested him. He'd heard, read, and experienced it all before. A hundred times. A million times.

Something tugged at the edge of his mind. There was a tiny upwelling, a renewal of a link to a consciousness he'd not felt since...since the last epoch of the godswar. Since before he'd gone into hiding. From his days as the divine artificer. The Maker.

"That cannot be." He closed his eyes and probed the source, shocked to find a vast well of *void* under a shell of *life* and *air*. A shell he had built. "The *Word of Xal* still exists. How? And why is it activating now?"

Inura suppressed his first instinct, which was to translocate directly to the source of the signal. That would have fit with his old body, his old level of power. But he was fragile now, and would make a tempting target for any god desiring the sudden acquisition of a vast reservoir of *life* magic.

He sketched a series of sigils artfully in the air, using the old style, the style that Xal had taught him. It didn't change their power, but it made them more elegant. It made the spell more beautiful and made the universe rejoice, as creation valued perfection wherever it was found.

A rippling mirror of flame bisected the air before him. Its milky surface resolved into an unfamiliar system, one with a tame yellow star and a single notable world.

That world was in the final stages of dissolution, something Inura had witnessed many times over his life. Gods were petty creatures, and knocking over another god's blocks, so to speak, was a common tantrum.

One Nefarius had brutally demonstrated upon the world Inura had invested the most heavily in. The only world he'd ever allowed to bear his name. But that was in the past.

The relevant question was...who had toppled *this* planet and why? He shifted the mirror's perspective, and it focused on a glittering fleet of derelict ships around the world.

The *Word of Xal* lay among that fleet, and she was not the only Great Ship. Others were there as well, whether dead or alive, and some remnant of what they were must have survived.

Hot, wet tears drifted into space, instantly crystalizing to ice. Inura thought he understood what might have happened here. When the battle had occurred, when Shaya had run with the *Spellship*, they'd all assumed this part of the Vagrant Fleet had been destroyed.

"How could I have been so blind?" Inura shook his head. He was so angry. Furious, even. At himself.

No longer was he the callous god he'd once been. In transferring his consciousness to his shade, he had absorbed that shade's memories. He'd seen what it was like to be mortal, and relatively powerless. It had become much more difficult to think of worshippers as currency.

He'd abandoned these people. When he'd thought the

ships dead he knew that a few Outriders and a handful of hatchlings had survived, but none of his children. No Wyrms.

And so he'd dismissed them. He'd watched a cloud of escape pods racing for the surface, and abandoned what he thought to be a dead fleet. Only it wasn't dead. Somehow the vessel's last captain, mighty Kemet, his great-great-grandson, a mere hatchling, had found a way to fool them all.

That raised a troubling question. If Kemet had saved the *Word* had he also found a way to save Ardaki? The staff had been thought lost, leaving Ikadra the sole key.

Only then did Inura see the ship clinging to the *Word*'s hull, a tiny white parasite with elegant curves, and enviable engineering. The result of his wayward children, who'd been co-opted by his enemies long ago, after their great betrayal.

The Inuran Consortium honored his legacy of artificing, and nothing else. They were thugs and bullies, and it didn't surprise him in the least to find them near such an atrocity. The idea that they might be allowed to seize control of the *Word* was unthinkable.

The Consortium might be able to wake the other Great Ships as well, which would make them a formidable power in the sector once more. They would use Inura's legacy to subjugate and exploit.

He could not allow it.

Yet what was the safest course? He was no war god to ride in and assault his enemies. He was a builder. A Maker.

He scanned the system for evidence of whoever'd done this, and it didn't take long to find the small Inuran fleet hovering over the doomed world like a drakeling waiting for prey to die.

Jolene would be in there somewhere; of that he was certain. He'd never met the woman personally, though he'd spoken with her daughter, Voria.

Did she still possess the Blood of Nefarious? If so, she could be a formidable opponent in his diminished state. He couldn't risk it. What if Talifax lived, and she served him? No, even coming here was a risk.

Yet he wouldn't leave without some small atonement. Inura scanned the world, and found a bright magical resonance on the southern continent. The spell emanated from a temple, a magical university in the old style, a beautiful stepped ziggurat that served as both a center of worship and learning.

The mages sheltering there likely had no idea of its significance. They'd forgotten why it was important, forgotten the culture that had given them birth, yet still they kept their charge. Still they clung to their honor, trying to defend that which they'd been charged with protecting.

Within their hallowed temple he sensed power. There were a number of potent artifacts, though in his estimation the real treasure were the thousands of mages desperately clustered around their temple.

Their collective magic channeled all eight aspects into a ward designed to hold their planet together as long as possible. It slowed the tidal forces, though the spell couldn't halt them. Their efforts might buy them a few more hours, at best.

Their loyalty must be acknowledged, even if it couldn't be rewarded. He could feel the Heka Aten connected to the *Word*. If the ship could be harnessed, then it was possible these people could be saved.

But only if the person taking the ship had time to forge the link. Time he could give them.

Inura raised both hands and began to sketch. His hands moved faster than the mortal eye could follow as he fashioned sigils together. In moments he held a spear twice as long as he was tall.

He flung the spear at the world, and watched as it sped toward the temple. In moments it vanished from sight, but as it impacted with the ziggurat he could feel his potent spell doing its work. The wards were strengthened. The disintegration slowed. It wasn't much, but it was as much as he dared risk.

Would that he were brave enough to reveal himself to his children.

26

T he flight back to the *Remora* was made largely in silence. We'd had our asses kicked, and Arcan had paid the price. I noticed that Rava was beginning to flag, and moved to take Kurz from her.

The weight on my shoulder was unfamiliar, but the unconscious man had a light frame. My newfound strength might have been enough to handle it, but I channeled an infuse strength anyway and then hurried up the corridor again.

It took maybe fifteen tense minutes to reach the ship, during which the red dots scurried around the bridge like ants. They didn't leave it or venture anywhere else in the ship, though some of them did disappear into the Inuran vessel. Probably to get more men and material.

Despair weighed on us all, from Briff's drooping tail, to the tears Rava was angrily trying to hide. Only Vee seemed unaffected, though I suspect that was more a function of her stoic mask than anything else. But then, what did I know?

I breathed a genuine sigh of relief when we collapsed at

the ramp leading into the *Remora*'s cargo bay. I gently set Kurz down, then sat heavily as everyone else did the same.

"I have a little strength left," Vee said as she finally broke the silence. "I will tend to my brother. I can wake him, at least. He's not seriously harmed." She moved to crouch next to us.

Rava and Briff were chatting in low tones while not paying much attention, but I couldn't have been more interested. It wasn't often you got to see *life* magic at work, and I was eager to study it when it wasn't being used directly on me.

If you took all the trappings away, that was what I loved most...magic. Learning about it. Using it. Understanding it. And I desperately needed some of that wonder right now, in the face of what we were dealing with.

Vee raised her hand to her brother's brow, and tenderly swept aside his bangs. She pressed her palm flat against his forehead, and closed her eyes as she began to hum a wordless tune.

Blue runes flared on her bracelet, and golden light pulsed from her palm into her brother. Kurz's eyes immediately fluttered opened, and he looked around him in shock.

"What happened?" He rose to a sitting position, and scrambled back a pace from his sister as he took in the room.

"You suffered a head blow when we crashed," she explained as she slowly rose to her feet. "I've relieved the pressure on your brain, which is why you woke up."

"Thank you." He rubbed at his forehead, then licked his lips. His beard still had flecks of blood and soot in it, and a small patch on the right side had been burned away. "What now, Captain? Do we flee?"

"That's on the table," I decided aloud, but then I shook

my head. "I haven't given up yet, though. Get up to the mess, grab some food, and catch your breath. I'll see if I can brainstorm a plan."

The whirring of my father's hoverchair heralded his arrival, and he appeared above the ramp, peering down at our ragged position from the *Remora*'s cargo hold. "Jer?"

"Hey, Dad. It didn't go well." I started wearily up the ramp, and clapped him on the shoulder as I reached him. "You were wrong about Arcan. He came through when it mattered."

"Oh." My dad's eyes grew wet, and he cleared his throat gruffly. "It's nice when people surprise you in a good way. There's no chance he survived?"

"There's every chance," I admitted, though I wished I didn't have to in front of Rava. In front of my sister. "They may want a prisoner to interrogate, and if they do there's a chance we might get him back. But let's be real, guys. It's unlikely." I turned around, and faced the others, who were all climbing the ramp. "We'd have to get on the Inuran ship, assuming it even stays put and that he's alive. We need to focus on taking the bridge."

I headed for the mess at a brisk walk that allowed a gap to form between me and the rest of my squad. They chatted softly amongst themselves, which left me a few minutes to come up with some sort of plan. If I couldn't, then we'd need to bug out, and the academy and all those cadets were history.

Once I entered the mess I flopped down in a seat at the table furthest from the door. As expected, when the others filed in they all sat at the opposite end of the mess. All except Vee, who moved to sit with me.

"May I join you?" she asked, nodding at the seat next to me.

I nodded wordlessly to it. She couldn't read my expression as it was behind my helmet, which I needed up if I was going to both monitor the enemy and talk to the ship.

Vee sat and rested both calloused hands on the table. The elegant bracelet was so at odds with the rough-spun clothing and the simple auburn ponytail. "You realize we're going to have to flee."

"Maybe." I squeezed the edges of the chair I was sitting in. I don't know why. A sudden anger surged through me, and bile rose in my throat. "Maybe not, though. You can sit here if you'd like, but I need a minute to talk to the ship. If I can't figure out a way to assault their position, then we'll pull out."

She nodded, and leaned back in her chair. Vee always had a patient air about her, and it calmed me. I liked that. I liked the casual murder vibe less so, but hey, we've all got flaws.

I cleared my throat, and addressed the ship. "Guardian, you said that I don't have access to the weapons systems, right?"

"Affirmative." The hatchling appeared in my field of view once more, complete with that amazing silver staff, tipped with a flying dragon.

"How about life support? Can I turn that off on their level?"

"Negative." The Guardian watched me expectantly.

How best to proceed? Vee was staring at me, but had remained silent.

I sat up straight as I had a sudden idea. "What systems do I have access to?"

"Propulsion, navigation, internal temperature and gravity, and all relevant subsystems." The Guardian smiled, which surprised me as I was beginning to think of this thing as a computer. "I am intrigued. It will be interesting to see if you can concoct a plan to dislodge them with the limited resources at your disposal."

"Them?" I asked.

"The group on the bridge," the Guardian explained. "Their armor and weapons are strange, but greatly reminiscent of Inura the Maker, and their magic does fit that conclusion. They have attempted to gain control of the ship, but their candidate was...insufficient."

"Insufficient?" I asked, now intensely curious. "What kind of trial is involved? I assume if you pass, you gain control of the ship?"

"Precisely." The Guardian nodded sagely. "If you pass the captain's trials—the trial of strength, the trial of reason, and the trial of judgement—then you will be declared the captain of this vessel until you declare another. We will be bonded. However, failure is terminal, as the last candidate learned to their detriment."

"That's interesting, but doesn't solve my problem." I tried not to stare at Vee, though I wasn't sure why I was smuggling glances when she couldn't tell if I was staring or not. "Let's get back to those systems. You said I have control over internal temperature and gravity, right?"

"Indeed." Guardian nodded, then gestured at the ship with his staff. "With level two control you can tend to the immediate comfort of the crew. Since this vessel wasn't created with a specific species in mind, you can tailor the atmosphere and gravity however you see fit. However, I cannot allow any action which will directly harm the occupants of the ship, unless ordered to do so by a captain."

"I see." A grin spread across my face. "Guardian, do you have a record of every species that has dwelled on this ship?"

"Of course." He gave a small indignant huff.

I already knew the answer to the next question, but I asked it in a way that would make it clear to Vee what I was getting at. "And you could, say, set the gravity on the bridge to match the requirements of any of these races?"

"Indeed." Another nod.

"How does the heaviest gravity ever used compare to the current gravity?" I'd guess our current gravity to be about 0.8 of normal.

"The Osmandi used a setting 324% higher than the current setting." The Guardian cocked his head. "This setting will not be immediately lethal to your species, though it will make it impossible to move under your own power, and prolonged exposure could be fatal."

"I'm aware of the risks. So I can order you to utilize the same gravity settings as the Osmandi?"

"Indeed." The Guardian offered another sage nod.

"Hey, Briff," I yelled across the mess. He and Rava glanced up from the conversation they'd been having on the far side of the mess. Kurz was sitting with them, though he didn't seem to be contributing much. I ordered the helmet to slither off my face so he could see my smile. "I've got a plan I think you're really going to love, and you get to be the linchpin. We're about to take this ship back from these bastards."

27

Threaded be the beauty of being captain, I found, was that you could just issue orders. I didn't have to explain the plan beyond telling Briff his part. I'd be doing the rest. So I assembled our ragtag squad at the base of the ramp in a rough line.

Briff stood in the center, his wings still shredded, but tail held proud. He cradled his spellcannon in both arms, and rested the butt unapologetically atop his belly.

Rava stood to his right. She'd fetched a sniper rifle from somewhere, something with a big caliber from the look of it. She'd only have to use it if something went wrong, but something going wrong was sort of our thing and I wanted us covered.

My dad floated on his hoverchair with a basic spellpistol cradled in both hands. I'd never seen him look uncomfortable, and he scrubbed a hand through his thinning hair as he looked around the hangar. He'd come, though, and hadn't questioned any of my orders.

Vee and Kurz looked the most relaxed. Kurz had wrapped a bandolier of vials over his shoulder, and each contained, if I understood correctly, a soul. How or why those were useful wasn't clear, but hopefully he surprised me.

Vee had a spellpistol belted to one thigh, and now carried one of Arcan's assault rifles. Being a mage, that meant we weren't making full use of her talents, but we didn't have another spellrifle to give her unless we wanted to ask the Inurans very nicely if they'd give us back what we'd lost in the crash.

It would have to do.

"Okay, let's move out. Vee, I want you on point, and I'll back you up." I moved into position next to her. "Kurz, follow a few meters behind us with Rava, and Briff will bring up the rear."

Vee started up the corridor and raised the hand with the bracelet, which flared briefly. A tiny white globe zipped playfully into the air over her head and raced up the corridor.

It illuminated a dozen meters in all directions, but the light was soft enough not to blind. Handy.

I admired the way Vee walked, both in the way a dirty mind might conjure and in a professional sense. She kept the rifle cradled loosely in both hands. It was ready to be brought up, but easy to carry until it was needed. Her head also scanned the corridor ceaselessly in exactly the kind of way I'd seen my father do when he ran point.

"Where were you trained?" I asked quietly. We had a few minutes walk, so I figured why not.

She glanced at me in clear confusion, and didn't speak for several more meters. Finally Vee glanced over her shoulder, at her brother, I realized, then back at me. "We do not speak of the Maker's Covenant with outsiders. My brother has already pressed the boundaries of what is permissible, and will likely face judgement if the elders learn what he has done."

I found myself smiling at her scandalized expression. "I was just working up to asking you out for coffee, not stealing state secrets. If you can't share your past, that's fine. I just feel like we have a lot of common ground."

"Is this really the right time to initiate courtship?"

"Uh, we're going to be dead in twenty minutes if this doesn't work." I raised an eyebrow in her direction. She hadn't relented. "Okay, fine, no more mating displays."

"Until after the op." She gave me something approaching a smile, then quickened her pace.

Was that flirting? Man, I was bad at this.

We continued in relative silence, which was broken by Rava and Briff retelling their comp stomp stories. That meant a lot, I think. They weren't focusing on Arcan's death. They were ready to fight. To get some payback.

My father, on the other hand, looked increasingly nervous the closer we came. I realized it might be a problem, and that it was my job to deal with it.

I trotted up alongside Vee. "I'm going to go talk to my father for a bit. Keep moving."

She nodded and did as I asked, the soft glow staining her hair into smoldering flame, which added to her ferocity.

I slowed my pace until my father drew even, then nodded in his direction. He nodded back while eyeing me suspiciously.

"You're worried about me," he accused as he raised his free hand to scrub his stubble. "I don't blame you. Not sure I still have this in me, kid."

I eyed him and tried to determine what the root cause was. I couldn't, so I asked. "So you can't hit targets?"

"No, my aim is good, I think. Not as fast as it used to be,

but I'm a good shot." He looked down at his pistol in disgust. "I will admit that this piece of garbage is part of the problem."

"If my plan works," I pointed out, "then it won't matter. You can pick up Ariela from whichever Inuran took her as a trophy. And if not, I'm sure they've got plenty of nice spellpistols to choose from."

My dad barked a short laugh, then shook his head as we continued up the corridor. "I never thought I'd be back at it, but now that I am I can't remember why I ever left it. I should have gone out with a gun in my hand a long time ago. Thank you for giving me a chance to do that. Whatever happens, I'm proud of you, son."

He zoomed a little closer, and wrapped an arm around my shoulder. My father was hugging me. A hug he'd initiated.

"Are you crying?" My dad demanded. He zoomed back like he'd been stung.

"No." And I totally wasn't. Okay, I totally was, but I, like... hid it. Okay, I didn't hide it. I was positive Vee'd seen, and probably her hawk-eyed brother had too.

Rava and Briff were still chatting, of course. I was going to have to separate those two during ops. Assuming we survived this one.

"We're getting close," Vee called softly from the head of the column.

I nodded at my dad, then willed the helmet to slither over my face. The HUD sprang up, and confirmed that none of the red dots had moved. They were dug in, ready to ambush anything that approached through the same corridor we'd used before.

"Guardian," I called, then paused until the hologram

appeared in my HUD. "There you are. Do you have a first name?"

"As a mortal I was designated Kemet, Admiral of the Vagrant Fleet." The hatchling stepped forward and thumped his holographic staff against the ground, which sent up a spray of illusionary sparks.

"Wait, Kemet as in the name of our planet?" I blinked at the hologram, and made some connections.

"Possibly." The hatchling shrugged, then fluffed his wings. "I do not know your history, though I can tell you of mine, if you require."

"Later," I promised, and meant it. I was going to spend so many hours picking this guy's brain. "For now, let's initiate my requested changes. Increased gravity in specified sections of the ship, then I'd like access to any internal cameras."

That last part had just come to me, and I was glad it had. I hadn't really considered how I was going to confirm that our plan had even worked.

"Immediately." Kemet tapped the staff again, and more sparks flared. It was like a punctuation mark. I kind of liked it.

A moment later my HUD flickered and an image appeared. It showed the room we'd fought in, which still bore scars from the combat. The remains of the rover were right where we'd left them, though if Arcan was dead, they'd definitely removed the body.

The Inuran troops were arrayed in a horseshoe formation behind barricades. Trios of snipers waited in the corners of the room, all focused on that one point.

A deep subsonic thrum pulsed through the room, and as it rippled over the defenders they simply collapsed to the deck. Every part of their body lay pinned however they fell, and not a single defender rose.

I began counting under my breath, and waited until I'd reached a hundred before taking another action. Not a single defender had reached their feet.

"This feels way too easy," I admitted, then turned back to the rest of the squad. "I can't see any problems though. Briff, you're up."

"A moment," Kurz called. He approached the hatchling, though he didn't look up from the deck. Then, in an instant, his entire demeanor changed. His posture straightened, and he rose to his considerable height. His eyes flared with a sharp sapphire light, the same that had come from Vee's bracelet. He carefully withdrew one of the vials from the bandolier, this one a sickly green color, then crushed it in his hand.

The smoke boiled out and coalesced into the same warrior we'd killed with the rover, though she now wore spectral versions of her armor and weapons.

Kurz raised a hand and pointed at the corridor ahead of him. "Steal the breath from any man in that room bearing this sigil on his armor, save the commanding officer." He indicated the Inuran logo on the spellpistol belted to his side.

The specter, or ghost, or whatever it was, nodded once, then flowed up the hallway.

"She's, like, not going to attack me, is she?" Briff asked as he shifted from scaly foot to scaly foot.

"Quite the opposite," Kurz assured the hatchling. He blinked a few times and the sapphire disappeared from his eyes. "She will do most of your work for you. For all intents and purposes, she will stop their hearts, one by one. Briff will be free to make his way to the commander, who should be wearing armor like Jerek's."

I didn't like the specter or the way being around it made me feel, and I was glad it had departed. Its use made me eye Kurz in a new light. I'd never encountered magic like his, and if it existed on Kemet, I'd never seen it in a holo or historical tome.

"You heard the man, Briff. Should be safe. We have a job to do. Find the person in the armor like mine, and bring them back here, dead or alive." If we obtained another suit that would dramatically increase our chances of survival, and who knew what other powers someone else could unlock?

Briff started up the corridor, and I followed him on the internal cameras. Briff passed the ranks of prone Inuran soldiers, and instead continued up the corridor to the door leading to the bridge.

It opened at the hatchling's approach, which seemed odd until I remembered the systems a level 2 had access to. They couldn't even lock the doors. They didn't have any more power than we did, despite having been here for days, weeks, or even months.

Briff walked into the bridge, and the image shifted to show him in the new room. That bridge contained, thank the maker, a recognizable spell matrix, which is what we used to magically power ships.

The device was made from three concentric rings. The first was forged from gold, the second silver, and the third bronze. Each ring rotated around the mage in the matrix, who had a stabilizing ring at waist height in case the ship takes a hit. Each ring was covered in sigils corresponding to the Circle of Eight, and by tapping them a mage can cast spells through the vessel itself.

Amazing.

Briff lumbered over to a figure in familiar Heka Aten armor who lay prone at the foot of the matrix. Eight guards lay scattered about the room in what would have been a perfect ambush pattern.

The hatchling crossed the last few meters, and then carefully picked up the commanding officer.

As he began to return, I caught a flash of green smoke rising from the mouth of one of the guards. It flowed into the next, exactly as Kurz had ordered.

I shivered, unable to savor the victory.

28

Briff dumped the commander's armored body unceremoniously at my feet. The entire squad had him covered, and I knew from experience that while the Heka Aten armor is cool...it doesn't make you invincible.

"Take the helmet off," I ordered as I jerked my pistol in her direction. "Make no sudden movements."

The helmet slithered from a handsome angular face framed by coifed platinum hair, and I got to observe the process from the opposite side for the first time.

That classic Inuran beauty was marred though, by a face made for sneers.

It wasn't sneering now. The blood vessels in both eyes had popped into a ghastly scarlet, and a trickle of dark scarlet blood leaked from one nostril. Gravity can be a real bitch.

"H-how did you manage to control the sh-ship's weapons?" He clutched at his chest, and I wondered how much damage the increased gravity had done. Part of me felt bad, though I didn't know why I should have.

I leaned in close, and tried to look menacing. He had to recognize my armor, and with my faceplate up maybe I even managed intimidating. "You're a little late for that information to be useful."

"Still," the Inuran rasped, "I wish to know. I do not understand how you bested us. Who are you? Did Voria send you?"

"Maybe." I had no idea who this Voria was, and filed that away for later. I leaned in a bit closer. "Why haven't you taken control of the ship?"

The man sneered, this time at himself. "I am weak. I was afraid to do what must be done, and sent underlings instead. They failed, and I squandered my chance. Now, please, tell me. Who are you? I cannot be told prior to my demise?"

I leaned back, and considered the question. Vee shifted behind me, which gave me an idea as to the next question I wanted answered. "How long have you been manipulating the lurkers?"

"Why does that mat—"

I impressed myself with how quickly I cocked the gauntlet into a firing position. The man's eyes narrowed. "You've puzzled out how to use the armor as a weapon, haven't you?"

"I have." I summoned a bit of *fire*, enough to make my fist glow white hot. "My patience isn't infinite. I have a disintegrating planet to deal with. If you aren't going to answer my questions I have a way around that. Kurz, get over here."

The lurker seemed surprised by my sudden attention. He stroked his beard as he crept over, almost a scuttle. His fear seemed directed at the Inuran, and I got the sense it was a personal sort of fear. He knew who this guy was.

"See those bottles?" I jerked a thumb at the phylacteries

in Kurz's bandolier. "Each one of those is a soul. Earlier you probably saw one of those souls tearing apart your goons."

"So you've recruited a soulcatcher." The Inuran rolled his eyes. "How exciting for you. We've eliminated all we could find. This one must have kept the practice secret. Always living in fear. Is that the way of it, urchin?"

I stepped between them and broke their line of sight. The Inuran looked up at me, the sneer firmly in place. So I punched him. Hard.

I don't know why I did it. Something broke inside me, a dam holding back all the frustration and anger I'd felt at every bully I'd ever dealt with, or who'd ever victimized my friends. This guy represented them all.

My fist crashed into his face, and his nose broke with a sickening crack. His bloodshot eyes narrowed into hideous pools, and he snarled wordlessly up at me.

"You work for Matron Jolene, don't you?" That was the name my mother had dropped, the Inuran head honcho. It made sense given their weaponry and accents.

"Of course not." He gave me a satisfied smile that exposed bloody teeth. "I acted alone. I am not part of any organization. Kill me if you like. Take my soul even. A barbaric act, and one that we put aside generations ago. But then...you are nothing if not barbaric, aren't you? You don't even know where your people come from, or who you were."

Were there other questions I could be asking? Maybe, but none leapt to mind. This guy had failed to control the ship, so what could he really offer? That meant we didn't need him.

"Kurz, you recognize this man, don't you?"

"Yes," Kurz whispered. He took a step backwards, and his gaze found the deck, but his voice remained strong.

Angry even. "He came to the first 'clave. He was the one who brought the gear they bribed us with. He was the one who convinced them all to go along with it."

"Well, not all of them, to be sure." The man seemed very satisfied for himself given his physical condition. "Some refused, but they've wisely scuttled from our sight. So long as they haven't interfered with the *Word of Xal*, we saw no reason to exterminate them yet."

"Yet?" Vee thundered. She lunged at the Inuran and caught him with a vicious backhand that snapped his neck back. "You were going to wipe us all out, weren't you? Genocide."

I recoiled at the slap, and something unpleasant fluttered in my stomach. I hated seeing this kind of wanton violence, much less participating in it, justified or not. Shooting someone was one thing, but inflicting pain...it just felt wrong. I hated what I'd just done with the punch. That didn't mean I couldn't be pragmatic though. I'm not stupid. Leaving enemies alive is always a bad idea.

"Vee, put him out of his misery. I'm going to head for the bridge." I rose and turned from the Inuran. I knew she'd have no problem dealing with the situation, but that didn't mean I wanted to be around to see it.

My father's hoverchair whirred closer and he delivered a concerned look. "It isn't easy, ordering your first death. You had to do it. You know that, right?"

"Yes," I snapped, hating the truth. "If we let him live, he's a threat and he could escape. If we let him go, he's an even bigger threat. We can't learn anything, so the only smart choice is..."

"...Hard as scales to make yourself do." My dad barked a self-deprecating laugh. "I hated it. I hate even seeing it. Better you than me."

"Yeah." I glanced at the bay where we'd increased the gravity, and on the other side where the bridge lay. "I'm going to head in there. Kemet, can you return the gravity to the previous setting?"

"Of course." The holo-dragon appeared in my field of view, and I earned another staff sparkle. "Done."

I walked through the bay and tried not to look at the bodies all around me. We'd killed them all without mercy or hesitation. Sure, they'd have done the same to us, but I hadn't had a lifetime to develop those instincts. It hit me harder than I'd thought it might.

Reaching the bridge made it easier to focus on other things. There were fewer bodies, thankfully, but that wasn't what took my mind off the carnage.

This was ancient magitech. Not just magic. Not just tech. This was the hybridization of both. We'd long since lost the secrets to forging it, and to my knowledge no one on Kemet had done any R&D for centuries.

The walls were a simple unadorned metallic purple. As I walked by, though, I made out faint black sigils flowing over the surface. The only other features of note were the breath-taking spell matrix and an arched doorway on the far side of the room, which was currently sealed with a black door.

I faced Kemet, which centered him in my HUD. "I take it that I need to go inside that door to face these trials you mentioned?"

"Indeed." No staff sparkle this time. "You can initiate the trials whenever you wish."

"Yeah, no." I loosed an unexpected laugh, and it felt good. "I'm more of a read-the-manual kind of guy. I want to know all about the trials before I go inside, and I want everyone else around to hear it." I activated the comm and sent the message to the squad, who'd yet to enter the bridge. "It's clear. Get in here quickly so we can seal this place."

Seal this place.

I shot to my feet and spun around, one gauntlet aimed in each direction. "Guardian, the Inurans attached a ship to the hull. That looks like it should connect to this location. Where is their point of entry?"

"Four meters to your left," Kemet supplied. He pointed the staff's outstretched tip toward the wall to indicate the location. "They are using an illusion to cloak their entry."

Anything could, and probably did, lurk beyond the illusionary wall. Who knew how many battle-hardened Inuran mages were waiting to renew the assault? I had to know.

I slowly approached the illusion, then leaned closer until my faceplate nearly touched the "wall". I rippled through like passing through water, and found a pair of Inuran mages staring right back at me a few meters up the docking tube.

Both carried spellrifles, but their posture was relaxed, and one of them even had the helmet of his spellarmor off. That armor was different from the others. More advanced. Newer. Inuran Mark IX maybe? I hadn't seen that model.

The moment they saw me I knew I was dead. I could probably drop one of them as they weren't prepared. But both? Not likely. I had to try.

"Officer!" the mage with his helmet still on hissed, then immediately snapped to attention.

The other mage's face melted into growing horror, like he'd done something monumentally stupid.

And then it hit me.

They didn't know. They didn't know their commander was dead. They didn't know their whole platoon was dead. These guys had been left behind to guard the ship.

And I was wearing identical armor to a man they feared.

I thought back to the Inuran, his manner, and his accent. I was pretty good with accents. One used what tools one had when at the academy and not terribly athletic.

"Incompetence," I snarled, and hoped that anything wrong with the voice would be associated with the armor. "You. If you cannot be prepared for battle, then you do not deserve to be armed. Give me your rifle."

The mage handed his spellrifle—a very, very nice spellrifle—across without a moment's hesitation. My sister would love it. I took it as if it weren't the most expensive weapon I'd ever held, then gave a disgusted snort.

"Do not allow any personnel to enter the dreadnought for any reason, unless I return to get you." Then I turned and stepped through the illusion.

Showing my back to those mages was the hardest thing I'd ever had to do, but as the seconds passed neither followed me through. It appeared my ruse had worked.

We had until they wised up to figure out how to make this ship fly.

29

I t didn't take long for the rest of the squad to arrive. I gestured for them to join me on the far side of the bridge, away from the illusionary doorway. Even Briff took pains to be quiet, though I figured if the guards did hear anything they'd be too frightened to investigate.

"All right, everyone." I whispered. "Here's the deal. That section of the wall is an illusion, and behind it is the access tube to the Inuran ship. There are two guards and probably more inside the ship."

Briff darted a panicked look at the wall, but kept quiet.

My father gave a low, almost inaudible whistle, which gathered everyone's attention. "Is there a reason we haven't rolled a grenade through that doorway? Seems like it would solve the problem."

"Not if the problem is six more Inuran Marines," Rava countered in a fierce whisper.

"Let's get control of this ship before we worry about that one." I turned to face Kemet's holographic form. "Can you project yourself here so everyone can see you?"

"Of course. This is the bridge." Kemet tapped the deck

with his staff, and this time everyone got to see the staff sparkle. "I can manifest anywhere on the ship, but here it requires no magic."

"Is that..." Briff trailed off as his jaw fell open. "Whoah. Is this guy the ship?"

Kemet delivered a stately bow, which included his wings and tail. "Indeed, brother. You may address me as Guardian, or Kemet as the officer candidate has elected to do."

"Brother?" Briff blinked those slitted irises.

Kemet nodded. "You are a *life* Wyrm, as I was in mortality. We are kindred, bonded by blood and scale."

"Okay," Briff allowed. He glanced down at his gut in embarrassment, and then straightened, clearly self-conscious. "Nice to meet you, I guess?"

"Kemet," I began, as I knew time was short. "We need some answers, and quickly. You said I can try to become captain, right? And that I need to walk through that arch? What will happen then?"

"The trials will begin," Kemet explained. Staff sparkle. Man, this guy loved that thing. "Once through the door you will enter the ship's reactor, a sliver of the god Xal. It is immense power that will incinerate most who enter. The magic there will guide you through three trials. If you survive, then you will be granted command."

"Can you tell me any more about these trials?" I folded my arms in what I hoped was a judge-y way. "This is kind of nebulous. Do they have names at least?"

"The trial of strength, followed by the trial of reason, and finally the trial of judgement." No staff sparkle. In fact, Kemet looked uncomfortable in a very Briff-like way. "I can say no more."

"I guess that's fair." I turned back to the crew. "I'm going to walk through that door in a minute. Before I do I have some questions about this ship. Feel free to chime in with your own." I turned back to Kemet's expectant face. "Where did this ship come from? And the other dreadnoughts? And why were they abandoned?"

"The ships are more than mere vessels." Kemet raised his wings in a dramatic fashion. Staff sparkle. "The Vagrant Fleet was exiled from the Great Cycle, cast adrift to wander the many-verse. It has fragmented countless times and worn endless forms. In my epoch the heart of the fleet was the Great Ships. Eight vessels prepared by the Pantheon to enforce their will throughout the galaxy. Our empire stretched the length of the galaxy. There wasn't a star we hadn't mapped by the end of our reign."

Kemet's face fell. He shook his head sadly. "I have listened to your transmissions. I had hoped the attack here was an anomaly, but it seems the godswar ended in ruin for the dragonflights."

"Maybe," Rava broke in, then shook her head. "I don't think so, though. There's a show called *The Last Dragonflight*. That means there's at least one left. It's about Outriders and *air* Wyrms. Lots of 'splosions and honor duels. Good stuff."

"Encountering a surviving flight would be a true wonder." Kemet gave a draconic grin, and you guessed it... sparkle. "You have renewed my hope. Thank you."

"Kemet," I interrupted as I was painfully aware of the neighboring guards. "Why didn't your enemies take these ships centuries ago? Why didn't they wipe out my ancestors on Kemet?"

"I...well, that name is quite flattering." His chest puffed up, and the grin broadened to inhuman proportions. "The fleet survived thanks to me. You see, I was the admiral in charge during the battle. We were ambushed, but we managed to escape into the depths. They tracked us, and finally cornered us here. I knew our only option was to stand and fight. They were coming for Ardaki." He raised the holographic staff to indicate that it matched the name.

"Anyway," Kemet continued, "I knew that if they believed the ships lived they'd never stop coming. I ordered all ships to simulate a self-destruct. We burned off all available magical power, all at once, knowing that it would confuse their scrying. They would believe us dead. So long as we gave them no reason to suspect otherwise they'd never be the wiser. As my last act I ordered all ships to expend their available magic in what appeared to be a detonation. They believed we had been destroyed. Then, when I was sure the ruse was a success, I did what any captain, or admiral, would do. I merged with my ship, and became the new Guardian. Which is how you've come to meet me so many thousands of years after my death."

I hadn't noticed until now, but Vee's expression had grown increasingly stormy as Kemet spoke, and had now blossomed into full-on rage.

"Are you saying that the Maker is nothing but a...ship?"

"All mother, no." Kemet hissed laughter. "Inura, the Maker, is an ancient *life* Wyrm. But he, and every other god in the Pantheon, gave of themselves to make these vessels. The *Word of Xal* is not a figurative name. It is literal. These ships embody their gods and their magic."

I am a fully trained archeologist, with a real passion for history. I had no idea what pantheon he was talking about, but Vee clearly did. Somehow the lurkers had maintained a memory of the old ships, while the people on Kemet had not.

A clatter came from the illusionary doorway. Metal on metal...like someone dropping a helmet.

"We need to get moving," I hissed, almost inaudibly. "Take me into this chamber."

"Of course." Kemet disappeared and in the same instant the black door retracted into the wall. Beyond it lay total unbroken darkness. Lovely.

"Briff, Rava, set up overwatch on that illusionary door. Kemet can show you where. Vee, see what you can learn while I'm gone." I turned to face her, and while she couldn't see me through the helmet, I hope she heard it in my voice. "There's a real chance I may not make it. If I don't, there's a second suit of armor. You or your brother can use that to make an attempt."

Vee nodded. There was emotion in her eyes, but I didn't know her well enough to know what it was. She gave my shoulder a squeeze, then moved to join her brother.

"You turned out all right, kid," my dad said. He barked a laugh. "No goodbyes, Jer. Get in there and get it done. No excuses."

My dad was right. There was no need for words.

"Be careful in there, Jer." Briff clapped me on the shoulder as I walked by.

"Thanks, bud. Will do." I smiled at the arch, and then stepped through.

Icy numbness caressed every part of my body, even through the armor. It was like diving into a winter lake and swimming to the bottom...naked.

A red aura appeared around the paper doll on my HUD, and began to pulse angrily. A light shade of yellow appeared over the chest, then spread to the arms and legs. Yikes.

"The test of strength," I muttered to myself as I pressed into the darkness. I had both arms outstretched, and awkwardly fumbled my way forward. "What the depths does that mean?"

I figured you'd want to test a captain, but were they talking about physical strength? Probably not. I seriously doubted I was supposed to pick up a rock. Perhaps it more meant endurance? Perseverance? Surviving the darkness?

I knew time was critical, since the yellow had continued to spread, and the temperature continued to fall. I could see my breath now, and my teeth chattered painfully.

I started to trot, which was terrifying in complete darkness, as I could be running toward a cliff. But I needed to reach something, and quickly. This place couldn't be endless.

Red bloomed in the armor's chest, and began to spread to areas that were yellow. I couldn't feel my fingers, or toes, or nose, or...other extremities.

I ran faster.

...And then I entered free fall. I pumped my limbs, but neither arms nor legs touched anything. There was nothing but darkness in all directions. Even my HUD had begun to dim.

I was falling, I thought, but with nothing visible around me I had no context and my brain had no idea what to do with that.

So far this test sucked.

"Guardian, can you hear me?" I called as I twisted in a slow circle in an attempt to see something. Anything.

There was no response.

I continued to fall, and the paper doll slowly turned red. As it turned out there was a color past red. Black.

A weak chime came from the armor, a dying alarm that was fast running out of power.

I was going to die. There was probably a specific route I was supposed to follow, and instead I'd tumbled into the death pit. Well, that sucked.

Was there anything else I could try before the armor failed?

I didn't think there was, so I relaxed into it. A pretty lurker had sort of flirted with me. My dad had said he was proud. That was pretty cool. I'd done my best to get my friends to safety, and I could die knowing they'd make it out.

I'd done everything I could. I was at peace.

30

I wasn't dead. That didn't seem right. My eyes fluttered open, and my breath echoed in the helmet. The armor was intact. In fact, the paper doll showed no damage at all.

The darkness was gone.

I now lay on a marble floor in a large antechamber to someone's ridiculously opulent mansion. I flipped over, rose to my feet, and took a good look around.

Antechamber was right. I was in a sort of sitting room with archaic hovercouches, the kind that had been lovingly handcrafted from the finest Shayan wood, and then lined with ghost-tiger fur.

The walls had many wide windows open to let in a clean breeze that smelled of summer. Beyond those windows lay impossibly tall mountains that stabbed into the sky.

I passed a vase on a stand that was probably worth more than the *Remora*. I had no idea how old it was, but the iconography predated anything I'd been taught about.

Where was I?

"You have passed the test of strength." Kemet appeared

in my HUD as if summoned, and offered an extra-enthusiastic staff sparkle. "Well done. I am pleased to see our descendants have lost none of their ingenuity."

"Wait, so what part of falling down a pit demonstrates strength? That's a terrible name for this test." I was genuinely offended. Who'd designed this?

Kemet loosed a holographic laugh. "The strength we speak of is character, my friend."

I found myself laughing as well. It was good to be alive. "Then why not call it that? You people need better engineers."

"Perhaps. Luck with the second test, candidate."

And then he was gone again.

I continued into the room, past the hovercouches, and found a high arched doorway leading to another room. A chandelier floated in midair, with wispy little flames dancing artfully about to provide dancing shadows to the occupants of the room.

Those occupants were the weirdest thing since the dino-porn meme had hit the arena circuit. They weren't dragons. But they weren't humans either.

The pair sat across from each other at a table. The one on the right could have been mistaken for a human at first glance. Except that he had draconic wings and a tail. His long white hair was pulled into a ponytail, and he was focused on a game board on the table.

The man on the left had a deep purple-hued skin that matched the *void* sigils I'd seen on the bridge. A pair of horns curled from his forehead, like the rams in the mountains above New Cairo. He also had a tail and wings, but his wings were more bat-like, and his tail was more slender and ended in a sharp barb. His mouth was full of razored fangs, and the sight of him touched a primal fear nestled deep within me.

Neither appeared to see me.

I approached, but neither moved. Both stared at the board, and once I was certain they weren't going to leap up and attack I did the same.

"It's a Kem'Hedj board," I realized aloud. I willed the mask to slither off my face so I could inspect their positions.

I loved the game, and had since I was a kid. Each side places a stone every turn with the goal of encircling their opponent's pieces. Games could go on for years if both players agreed to expand the board.

The white player had a more defensive style. He advanced cautiously, instead choosing to fortify positions so they could not be assailed later. The black player was more aggressive, as fit his ferocious appearance. However there was a nuance to his play that suggested a mastery that vastly exceeded my own.

When I say my own, I suppose I should clear that up. I was good back at the academy. I used to clean up in the lounge for pocket money. But I wasn't amazing. I was just good enough that when the guy with real talent showed up, I stopped swaggering and started listening.

The game I was observing was the sort of thing that masters would spend years studying before finally puzzling out the winning move. There was no way I would suddenly manifest the ability to solve this.

I could experiment. Placing a piece could be trial and error, but I imagined something called the trial of reason would require a bit more reasoning. So how could I get the answer?

I sat down next to the table and reached into the side pouch on the armor. I'd stowed a couple of protein bars and was starting to feel the hunger. Who knew how long I'd been unconscious.

I unwrapped the bar and was about to bite into it when both wrapper and bar dissolved. Not the "it's an illusion" kind of dissolve either. I watched them disintegrate quite literally in my hands.

"Uh." I wasn't sure what the depths to do now. I couldn't eat? Maybe it was one of the rules. "Back to solving this I guess. Not much of a lunch break."

I rose to my feet and turned to the board again. And I got angry. "Guardian, if you're listening, your tests suck."

So I decided to cheat.

I raised my palm and grinned like a child who was getting away with something. I conjured the very same blue flame I'd used outside that armory what felt like a lifetime ago. I peered into its depths, and drew upon *dream* to peer into the past.

I scrolled backward, minute by minute, watching the game board change in the flames. That didn't get me very far so I moved to ten-minute increments. Then hour increments. Piece by piece, the game rolled back until the first white piece was placed.

Then I let it roll forward, and I studied the game play. I watched it unfold, and gawked at the mastery I was witnessing. These people were legendary, and would destroy any grandmaster back on Kemet. It was amazing.

Remember that cheating part? Flame reading doesn't just work on the past. It can project the future, which is why it is banned in all casinos, and casinos without magical protection aren't very profitable.

I let the game proceed, and the white player bent to add another piece. Then the black player. I watched the entire game play out. There were eleven more black moves and ten more white. I replayed the sequence three more times to be sure I had it perfectly, then I banished the flame.

I plucked a black stone from a golden bin and placed it where I'd seen the first stone placed. A chime sounded in the distance, and the white player bent to make his move.

It took a while to repeat the process, but after a few more minutes I reached the end of the sequence. The final move. I bent slowly, then paused long enough to summon my helmet again. Just in case.

I placed the last stone, and waited.

"I am impressed." Kemet appeared with a broad grin already in place, and this time I was treated to the coveted double staff sparkle. "Few candidates have ever made it this far. You will find the final test, the test of judgement, in the next room." The holo-hatchling pointed at the far side of the room, where I saw an open arch in the wall.

Had that been there before?

I supposed it didn't matter. I hurried through the door and into the final trial.

31

"Captain! Captain!" a woman shouted into my face. "What are your orders?"

Somewhere in the background a klaxon blared, and I realized I was standing on the bridge of the *Word of Xal* during the height of combat. The matrix was still there, but now the entire forward-facing wall had been altered to show the background of space.

I recognized Kemet in the distance. A whole, undamaged Kemet. I did not recognize the fleet of enemy ships closing on our position.

"Captain," the woman demanded again. "The black fleet has moved to engage, and the *Shivan's Echo* has already been disabled. What do we do?"

A slow smile spread across my face. This was basically a video game. I'm really, really good at video games, and I've sunk countless hours into all different sorts.

"Mark all enemy ships," I ordered, and gave a satisfied nod as a red triangle appeared next to each of the ships. "Display combat threat assessment on a scale of one to a hundred and tag each vessel."

The woman, an assistant I assumed, closed her eyes. Numbers rippled through the enemy fleet, and I could now see their capital ships, right down to their fighters, each with some idea of how powerful the ship was.

"Apply the same assessment to our fleet, and tag them accordingly." I moved to the spell matrix, and caressed the stabilizing ring lovingly. I'd always wanted to step into a real spell matrix, but truth be told, I'd only ever used the simulator at the academy.

I ducked through the slowly spinning rings, which made a faint *whum whum* as they rotated around me.

My fleet had now been tagged, and it became blindingly obvious that I was outnumbered and outclassed. They had more ships, and the computer had assigned them much higher numbers. Our fleet possessed eight great ships, each given a ten.

The lead moon-sized enemy vessel, the one I was concerned with, had a twenty-five next to it. Several smaller ships accompanied it, each with a crimson five.

"Concentrate all fire on the lead vessel. Ignore the smaller ones." I extended a cautious finger, and tapped the *fire* sigil on the bronze ring, then the silver, and finally the gold.

Wave after wave of potent flame rolled from my chest, falling to the floor and disappearing into the ship. Deep within the vessel something primal hummed, and the power I fed was amplified a million-fold.

"Main cannon ready, Captain," the woman who'd been yelling in my face supplied.

I tapped the *fire* sigils again, and the entire ship shook. A spear of divine fury, starstuff charged with the will of a god, hurled from our spellcannon. It streaked through the intervening space and slammed into the much larger enemy vessel.

The spell washed over the hull, and for a moment the enemy vessel disappeared from view. When it reappeared, the outer carapace had been singed, but nothing more.

"That's not encouraging."

I decided to wait for the rest of our opening salvo. Spells streaked from the other great ships, each slamming into the enemy in rapid succession. The acid bolt from the *Earthmother's Bulwark* did the worst damage, but it was the light bolt from the *Inura's Grace* that split the enemy vessel down its center. It detonated spectacularly, and took the smaller ships with it.

I pumped a fist in the air. Nice. "Order all vessels to fall back at half speed."

The blips moved on the screen, and the enemy fleet followed us closely. Several other rating twenty-five ships accelerated from the main body. We had better range, but they were much, much faster.

They were going to catch us eventually, and presumably their close range weaponry would be devastating.

"Uh, you." I pointed at the woman who'd been speaking to me. "What's your rank?"

"Adjunct, sir." She eyed me quizzically. "Are you all right?"

"Which one of our ships is the fastest?" I scanned the little tags, but they didn't seem to list speed.

"The *Virkonna's Saber*, sir," she supplied. "Shall I issue an order?"

"Have the *Saber* accelerate to maximum speed. Head for that planet's umbral shadow." I pointed at Kemet, though I suspected she wouldn't know that name.

The *Saber* almost immediately peeled off from the main fleet, and accelerated toward the Umbral Depths.

"All other ships," I ordered, "concentrate on the lead enemy vessel. Once it's down, hit the next."

As I'd expected, all four enemy ships were trying to cut off the *Saber*'s escape. They had to pass our position, which put them in range of multiple cannons.

The first of the four enemy vessels exploded under a withering volley of spells, as did the second. The third was severely damaged, but the fourth made it out of our range before we could finish it.

That last ship caught the *Saber* before it reached the umbral shadow. Hundreds of tendrils exploded from the black ship, and each latched onto the *Saber*'s silvered hull. They burrowed into the ship, and began eagerly devouring metal, crew, and magic alike.

The *Saber* was drawn inexorably toward the black ship's main body, where a massive tendril shot forth and impaled itself deep in the Great Ship's core. The *Saber*'s momentum died, and the power died shortly after. The enemy ship continued to feed, while its wounded brethren turned back in our direction.

We finished the wounded black ship easily as it approached, but there were many, many more waiting in the distance. They were closing on our position, and I didn't know how much longer we'd be able to keep out of range.

"I take it back," I muttered. "Not loving this test as much as I thought I would."

A dozen more enemy twenty-fives glided toward my fleet. They were going to be in firing range before we reached the umbral shadow and escaped into the depths.

"Adjunct." I cleared my throat as a sudden lump

appeared. My body was already judging me for what I was about to do. "Which Great Ship is the slowest?"

"The *Earthmother's Bulwark*." She cocked her head. "Why, sir?"

"Order them to move along a perpendicular course immediately."

"But, sir, the enemy will catch—"

"DO IT!" I thundered. Something broke inside of me. Something about this spell, whatever it was, had given me an emotional attachment to this fleet. They were my family, and I was killing them.

The *Earthmother's Bulwark* slowed, then turned at a sharp angle. Eight of the black ships made for it, and opened a large enough gap for the rest of the fleet to reach the umbral shadow.

"Have one of the ships open a Fissure." I rested against the stabilizing ring, wrung out and demoralized. "Order the rest of the ships to form up on our position, and follow the course we broadcast."

The sky beneath Kemet cracked open to expose the shadowy universe underlying our reality. We passed through that hellish portal, to the temporary safety of the Umbral Depths.

Guardian's form instantly appeared in my field of view, and if anything, his grin was even wider. "I can scarcely believe it."

"What?" I blinked up at him, the weight of the battle still crushing me.

"The intensity of the experience will fade," the hatchling promised. "You have passed the test of judgement."

"This time I get it. I wasn't the one being judged. You were testing my judgement."

"Precisely." There was the staff sparkle I knew and loved. "You made difficult choices to maximize the survival of your crew. That is the exact quality I seek in a captain. You have done well, and earned your reward."

32

The combat, the bridge, and my emotional connection to them vanished. There was a moment of darkness, and then I was elsewhere once more.

I stood in a vast chamber, the ceiling and walls disappearing into the darkness. The only illumination was a faint purple glow, which came from everything. The power of the *void*, I realized.

"Where am I?" I asked, unsure if my body could even make words any more.

A figure coalesced next to me. It began as a raw pool of purple magic, then molded itself into a tall, imposing body that loomed over me. Wings sprang from the back, and a tail, even as scales burst out to cover skin.

Once the process had completed I was starting at the Guardian. Not a holo. Not a representation. This was the real thing. The being itself.

"We meet at long last." Kemet extended a clawed hand toward me.

I took it, and shook. His palm was cool to the touch, and crackled with power. He released my grip, and extended a hand. Something glittering rose from the muck. A long, slender staff...with a dragon in flight at the tip. This was the real thing, not an image.

"Meet your charge, Captain." Kemet did not offer me the staff, but did hold it up for my inspection. "This is Ardaki, one of twin keys created to interface with the most powerful vessel in creation. I have safely hidden it here for countless millennia. We stand in the heart of the *Word of Xal*, in the pool of *void* magic gifted by Xal, and shaped by Inura the Maker."

I examined the staff closely, but didn't touch it. Immense magic pulsed from it. Many-layered multi-aspected magic of the type no mortal could shape on their own. This required teams of magitech engineers, backed by the raw power of a demigod, or possibly a god.

"I take it we should leave it here then? Removing it will make it possible to find?" I finally raised a hand and caressed the metal. It thrummed in my hand, begging me to take it up.

"Indeed. This is the only safe place. I do not know what became of the *Spellship*, but if it exists, and if Ikadra does not, then Ardaki will be the only means of controlling the vessel." He folded his arms and the staff descended back into the liquid magic. "There are many things to discuss, but I know you have a situation of some urgency. Full control of the vessel is yours. How do you wish to proceed?"

That was the real question. I rubbed at the back of my neck and stared up into the darkness at the faint purple glow in the distance.

"Let's start with diagnostics," I decided aloud, then faced

Kemet. "Does life support work, and if so, can we support, say, twenty thousand crew, comprised primarily of humans and drifters, with some hatchlings?"

"Indeed." Kemet raised a hand, and the magic coalesced into a cutaway of the ship. "Only these three areas are too damaged for life support to function. However, many secondary systems are in need of repairs, and we have no means of producing food."

"We can deal with that later, I suppose." I studied the model of the ship. "I guess my next question is what will it take to..." I trailed off as I realized the Inuran vessel was still attached to the hull. "Do we have a weapon system that can deal with that ship?"

"Negative. Internal defenses are inoperable." Kemet shook his head regretfully. "We lack sufficient power to fire the main spellcannon, though it wouldn't help in this instance."

"What do you mean?" I glanced at the hatchling. "How does power work in this vessel?"

"This is the main core." He gestured around him with both outstretched hands. "It is a vast reservoir of *void*, and over time it produces a...residue that the vessel funnels into all power systems. The core has been depleted for many centuries now. Jump starting it will require a significant infusion of magic."

"Hmm." I drummed my fingers along my pistol, and returned my attention to the cutaway of the ship that the Guardian had conjured for me. "We do have some limited power, right?"

"A small amount, yes." Kemet nodded, concern etched on his draconic features. "But the quantity will be fast burned away. If you do not use it to secure additional magic, this vessel will be unable to journey to your world. Your people will die."

"Well, crap." Another seemingly unsolvable dilemma.

The thing about unsolvable dilemmas is that they usually *are* solvable, but you lack the perspective or resources or time or knowledge to see the solution. "Can we scan the enemy ship any more successfully now that I have full control? I need to know how many people we're facing. Maybe we can overwhelm them, or dupe them. They might have something we can use. In fact, they must have if they were planning to restore the ship."

"Negative." Kemet shook his scaly head. "I can erect a forcefield around their means of entrance, but it will further deplete our reserves."

"Don't bother. There's no point in wasting the power. How long was I unconscious?"

"You were not." Kemet gave a low chuckle. "This is playing out in the space between breaths. To your companions you have just entered the mysterious darkness."

"Wait, so you're telling me that I actually have time to think through a solution? I can take a nap?" I gave a delighted laugh. It had felt for a while like things were never going to go my way again. That appeared to be changing. "Okay, so we need a source of magic or we're boned, right?"

"Affirmative, if by boned you are alluding to our slow and ignoble end."

"Yeah, you get it," I confirmed. I focused on the cutaway of the ship again, specifically on the Inuran cruiser. "Can you zoom in on their ship?"

Kemet raised a hand and the void energy rearranged itself into a closer view. The Inuran ship was all artful curves. Sleek and elegant. The white hull was a clear challenge. It said we aren't bothering to hide. Know that we're here, and tremble.

The Inuran Consortium was, as I'm sure you've gathered, the premier magitech artificing organization in the sector. Maybe in the galaxy. All their ships wove magic into everything from the hulls to the spelldrive to, morbidly, the mages who crew the ship.

See where I'm going with this?

"Kemet, this ship is *void*-aspected, right?" I was staring at the *void* all around me, so it was sort of an obvious question.

"Indeed." The hatchling cocked his head and watched me.

"We can use that to teleport the ship, right? Just like the blink spell, but for the entire vessel?"

"That capability exists," Kemet allowed. "However, it has never been employed. Generally we use *void* both to maneuver, through gravity magic, and to open a Fissure to enter the Umbral Depths. Direct teleportation is hideously inefficient from a magical sense, and we lack the power to move the entire vessel."

"Can we teleport other things? Smaller things. Like, say...that Inuran ship."

Kemet's slitted eyes widened, and then an unsettling smile bloomed. "Indeed we could. Where would you like to teleport it? Into the sun perhaps? That will ensure they are no longer a threat, and leave you free to solve the magic dilemma."

"The Inurans are the solution." My stomach roiled, and several thoughts flashed through my head. I saw the merc I'd melted. I saw myself walking away after ordering Vee to murder our prisoner in cold blood. Now, I was crossing the next line. I was going to kill a ship full of people, and I didn't even feel bad about it. What did that make me? "Teleport the Inuran vessel directly into the reactor."

"Are you certain?" Kemet's tail slashed behind him in agitation. "I have no idea what that will do."

"Let's hope my academy education was worth my mom's credits." I raised a hand and sketched a line in the cutaway of the ship Kemet had provided. "If we're here, and if this is pure *void* magic, then it will disintegrate anything it comes into contact with, right?"

"Presumably."

"And magic can neither be destroyed or lost. Merely transmuted or moved."

"Ingenious!" A grin enveloped Kemet's entire face, and he reached for a staff to do the sparkle thing. His disappointment at not being able to do it was palpable. "Ah, in any case, your idea has merit. Stronger magic will transmute sympathetic aspects into itself. If we teleport the ship into the reactor..."

"...It will digest the ship," I explained. "And the crew. And that magic, hideous as it is, might jump start the ship."

"Shall I proceed?" Kemet asked, his wings held high.

"Do it."

"Ah, one last thing," Kemet cautioned. "If you are successful in re-igniting the reactor it will also fully realize your link to the ship."

"I don't know what that means, but I guess I'll find out. Do it." I hoped I was doing the right thing. Of course, when you only have one apparent action, and inaction means everybody dies, it's hard to call it the wrong choice no matter how it works out.

The air around me vibrated, and all magical constructs, including the Guardian, melded back into the floor. I was alone for a just long enough to wonder what was happening, and then the air above me began to warp and fold.

The entire upper portion of the cavern was suddenly occupied by an Inuran cruiser, which looked even larger when you were standing underneath it. The massive white vessel began to fall toward me, and in a few seconds I was going to be crushed. There was nowhere to run. Nothing I could do to avoid it.

Purplish tendrils exploded from the walls, each wrapping around a part of the vessel. It was tugged in a hundred directions as ravenous tentacles tore pieces loose and dragged them back into magic. The feeding frenzy was disturbing, and the idea that I was participating in it left a disquiet residue.

It all happened so fast, and the only emotion that made it through the numbness was relief that I couldn't see any people aboard. I couldn't hear their screams. If they were there, like the guards I'd met, then they'd died quickly and silently.

The walls began to glow. The faint purple became a wild pulsing violet, and then the energy exploded from the walls...toward me. It washed over my armor from all directions, wave after wave after frigid wave.

The magic passed through the armor, through me, and out the other side. Each time a wave moved through, it became harder to breathe as the magic deposited something in my chest.

I fell to my knees and clutched at my heart, which no longer beat. My lungs worked furiously to somehow compensate, but black spots filled my vision.

Impossibly cold fury burst from my heart, and flowed up every last artery, every last neuron, every last cell. The *void* permeated all of me, to my very soul, and still it kept coming.

Eventually my awareness of the waves stopped, and a euphoric clarity overtook me. The universe stretched before me. There was Kemet, dissolving before my eyes. There, in the distance, was the Confederacy I'd heard so much about. Mighty Ternus, with their New Texas Military, and Colony 3, the breadbasket of the sector.

I could see Shaya, with its mighty tree, so tall it pierced the atmosphere. I could see Yanthara, and the fire god who slumbered there. I peered into the Erkadi Rift, where the Krox and Ifrit lurked.

I saw beyond our sector. Beyond our time. Beyond our reality. I was the past, the present, the future, the fractured realities of countless might-have-beens. I became the universe, for just an instant.

Then it all faded, and I was left gasping on the floor, too weak to even stand. At first, anyway.

I sat there panting, but after a moment I became aware that Kemet had returned.

"Well done, Captain." He placed a supportive hand on my shoulder, and gave a friendly squeeze. "The ship is yours, and ready for battle. In a limited fashion, of course."

"Yay," I rasped, utterly worn out. "Can you teleport me to the bridge?"

"Of course." He snorted a laugh. "But why not do it yourself?"

Only then did I realize that the *void* magic still dwelled inside me. It smoldered in my chest, just like *dream* and *fire*. *Void* was sharper. It required more precision. It was cold and brittle. But it was powerful, and now a part of me.

I closed my eyes and willed the ship to send me back to

the bridge. There was a brief moment of vertigo, and then I appeared standing next to the rest of my squad.

My father was the first to spot me. He'd been sipping a drink through a straw, but the straw tumbled to the floor forgotten. "Lady's big ole kitties, you scared at least ten years out of me. Where did you come from?"

"The core," I shot back with a grin. "I've dealt with the Inurans. How about we go save some people back on Kemet?"

33

I thrust out a hand toward the bridge's opposite wall, and willed it to transform into a viewscreen the same way I'd seen in the test. It worked! The wall shifted into a perfect view of the debris field around us, and in the distance I could see just how dire things had become for our planet.

"Whoah," Briff said. He walked over and placed a hand on the wall. "It's like touching the *void*. Awesome. You really are in control of this thing."

"You communed with a Great Ship," Vee said as she moved to stand before me. She cupped my chin in her hand and gently peered into my eyes. "I can see the *void* inside your pupils. It's like peering into the Umbral Depths. You've been marked by a god."

I nodded. She wasn't wrong, but I didn't have time to explore what that meant right now. Debris was flowing away from my planet at an alarming rate. I had to act.

"We need to focus on saving people." I pointed at my father. "Dag, I'm promoting you to sergeant. Rava, congrats, you just earned corporal. Briff, you report to Dag. Dag, take your people down to the aft cargo bay and get ready to receive a whole lot of very confused guests."

"Uh, sure, Captain." My dad was a wonderful blend of pride in his son and utter confusion. "What will you be doing?"

"I'm going to make the *Word of Xal* teleport the entire academy into the cargo hold." I explained it like relating the weather. "We're going to have a lot of scared, confused people. Most of those people will recognize your face. They know Dag the Slayer. You can keep those people calm."

"On it, Captain." My dad gave a loose salute, then zoomed over to door. "Come on, kids. We've got work to do."

"What about us?" Vee asked. She nodded at her brother. "We have skills that could be of use."

"This ship is on borrowed time." I saw no reason not to give it to her straight. "I jump started the core by feeding it the Inuran vessel. I'm pretty good at magical theory, and I've done the math. For me to get fifteen thousand or so kids and a lot of material teleported from the surface into our hold is going to bleed this ship dry. We'll be right back where we started...immobile without much other than life support."

Kurz and Vee exchanged a glance. Her expression promised swift death if Kurz broke some unspoken agreement. He did it anyway.

"Captain..." Kurz licked his lips, pausing to gather his strength before continuing. "Our people were given the secrets to maintaining these ships. We are descended from mechanics and engineers, from the people who built and maintained this fleet. If you are asking us to help you keep this one running, then I'd argue we have a sworn duty to do exactly that."

"Don't," Vee warned. Her eyes narrowed. "Not yet, Kurz. Not until we contact them."

"I would appreciate," I interrupted, "any help you both can offer me *without* betraying your people or your ideals. Keep this ship running, and your secrets are your own. Seem fair?"

"Deal." A smile ghosted across Vee's face. "I'll even call you Captain."

"More than fair, Captain." Kurz offered a grateful nod. "I will begin surveying power relays and searching for damage."

They filed off the bridge, which finally left me alone. I wanted my wits about me for this one, just in case my mother insisted I speak to the minster on the spot.

I moved to the spell matrix and lovingly caressed the stabilizing ring as I slipped inside. My matrix. My ship. It didn't feel real. Somehow I knew it couldn't last.

The rings slowly rotated around me with their faint hum. I tapped *fire* on all three, and a missive appeared on the wall I'd turned into a viewscreen. It took a moment to be accepted, but then my mother's face filled the wall.

"Jer?" Her eyes shone and I don't think she'd ever worn that large a smile in her entire life. "We scryed some sort of magical explosion in the fleet. I was hoping you were involved. Does this mean you're on that dreadnought?"

"It does," I confirmed, not wanting to leave her in suspense. "We have control of one of the Great Ships, Mom. It's called the *Word of Xal*. I have so much to tell you, but we can get to that later. I need to get down to the academy. We've got enough space in the hold to save everyone."

My mom blinked, unable to find words for several moments. "I...see. I don't know how you pulled it off, but I am amazed. Let me speak to the minister. I'll let her know you'll contact us once you've completed the evacuation."

"Uh, there's a reason I called you first." I inhaled slowly. I don't know why I feared telling my mother this. I wasn't a student any more. "The, ah, headmistress isn't overly fond of me. I still owe some fees, and we exchanged some words...a missive from the minister could go a long way to making sure this all happens quickly."

My mother's eyes narrowed and thunderclouds descended. "You are going to tell me this story once we have this situation under control. Don't think saving the academy will get you any slack, either."

"Thanks, Mom. I'll be in touch." Abort! Abort! "Love you."

"Love you too." There was no Jerbear, and the thunderclouds had only worsened by the time the missive disconnected.

The whole incident at the academy seemed so laughable in the face of imminent destruction. Maybe we focused on it because it was a way to pretend the situation wasn't happening. To be normal. Who knew?

"Guardian?" I called. I figured he was nearby, and I was right.

"Yes, Captain?" Kemet appeared before me with a holographic Ardaki in one hand.

"Let's work on some logistics." I nodded at the screen. "I want to retrieve an academy from the surface, buildings and all. How do I best go about that?"

"Mmm, this will require precision." A long tongue flicked over his teeth contemplatively. "Were it me, I would conduct a survey on the surface. This will allow you to specifically target whatever mass you wish to move. However, there is one further...complication."

"Of course there is." I suppressed an eye roll. "Elaborate."

"You will need a conduit to the *Word of Xal* to activate the teleport," Kemet explained. He nodded at Ardaki. "That means using the staff. With Ardaki you will lessen the magical requirements and increase the amount of mass you can move. As our magical reserves are critical, this seems a prudent risk."

"You said if we took it out of the ship, the bad guys would find it," I growled, quite aware of my accusing tone. "That sounded very, very bad. Is some angry god going to come after us? Am I going to have to deal with the hungry, hungry ships from the test of judgement?"

Kemet gave a helpless shrug, which involved his wings. "I do not know. It is possible. However, if you limit the time that the staff is out of the core, and if you are careful not to reveal to anyone what the staff is, you should be fine, I'd think. No one is likely to recognize it."

"Okay." I hated extra complications. "So, how do I get Ardaki?"

"Will it," Kemet supplied. "Nearly all command actions are initiated this way. Envision what you need, and it will become reality."

That sounded simple enough. I extended my right hand and envisioned the staff there. To my immense shock the air popped and folded, and the universe deposited the staff into my hand.

I could feel the intelligence within the silver haft. It wanted to be wielded.

"Well done." Kemet bowed. "Good luck in your mission, Captain."

Then I teleported down to my alma mater to save them from imminent destruction.

INTERLUDE VI

Jolene hurried to her desk and waved a hand over it as she approached. The surface sprang to life, and data populated all over the screen. She waved away notifications until the clutter was gone, then focused on the view itself.

Right now the desk showed the Great Ships, a view of all of them. Seven in total, though it was unrealistic to expect that all could be salvaged. That hardly mattered, though.

If she could salvage even three, her fleet would be one of the greatest powers the sector had ever seen. What's more, she'd have access to the knowledge of the ancients.

What clues had Inura inadvertently left behind? Their creator had finally revealed himself during the last Godswar, and had foolishly allowed himself to be slain. He was no more, squandered for no good reason in an endless cycle of war between gods.

She honored his memory, but did not miss him. She would make use of the knowledge that he'd left behind, and who knew? If *Inura's Grace* was among the surviving ships she might find a way to replace him.

A red exclamation point appeared on the screen, and she tapped it. It inflated into a graph with relevant information about a magical event that the flame readers had just detected with their scrying.

"This makes no sense unless they succeeded," she muttered, then pinched in the air near the screen to zoom in on the *Word of Xal.* The vessel leapt into clarity, and the moment she glimpsed the violet glow coming from the reactor and weapons, she couldn't help but grin. Her plan was finally coming together.

The *Word of Xal* was waking up.

She hardcast a missive, the *fire* and *dream* sigils fusing into a mirrored surface. Only...it wasn't mirrored. It was cloudy. That would only be possible if Valat was blocking scrying, which she wouldn't put past him...or if he was dead.

Jolene returned her attention to the *Word of Xal*, but this time she was scanning for her cruiser. White on black near the bridge should have been easy to spot, yet she saw nothing. She spent a good minute combing the image, but the ship was simply gone.

Ordinarily she'd trace it, but due to the secrecy of the mission, she'd shielded that vessel from scrying. The wards had been architected by better minds than hers, and there was no way she'd be able to pierce them. Not even with Inuran resources.

What did it mean? Had her underlings fled? That made no sense. Why flee when it appeared that they had somehow accomplished their mission? There were no scenarios that fit the facts.

None that she was ready to accept, anyway.

The screen's edge rippled red, and she accepted the incoming missive. It showed the sub-bridge where her subordinates took care of the day-to-day matters of the ship.

"Pardon, Matron," a blond tech of too few years bumbled out. "We deemed this matter urgent enough to interrupt you. We have just intercepted a missive between the *Word of Xal*...and the minister of Kemet."

"And?" she demanded. "What does it say? I want to hear this conversation. Now."

The tech squirmed uncomfortably. "We are not familiar with the modulation, and there are several layers of wards encrypting the communication." She blinked uselessly, clearly waiting for instructions.

"I will deal with it," Jolene snarled, then terminated the connection.

Who was in command of the *Word of Xal*, and what were they telling the minister? The most likely explanation was that she'd been betrayed by Valat, but that didn't feel right.

He had no relationship with the minister, and nothing to gain by communicating with her. Had he betrayed her, he'd have left the system.

That meant someone loyal to Kemet was in charge of the vessel, and if that was the case, it meant they might have the resources to unmask her. It didn't matter if they served Voria or Xal'Aran, or some other deity. They'd all crush her like vermin.

And that meant she had to leave. Not abandon her plans entirely, but certainly be elsewhere if and when her enemies arrived. There was still the plan with the majority vote, which she would soon have, thanks to Bortel. And even if that failed she'd inherit the fleet when the trade moon arrived and these unwashed mercenaries couldn't satisfy the contract they'd signed.

In all cases she won.

That was why she was leaving. Not because she was

afraid. She would go elsewhere to await final victory, secure in the knowledge that she had won.

34

I closed my eyes and took ten deep breaths. I figured I could spare that much time to center myself and get ready for what I was about to do. It wasn't just facing a headmistress who'd terrified me for five years. It was the knowledge that if I miscalculated, if I did something wrong, then some or all of these people would die.

It would be my fault.

As a card-carrying screwup I know what it's like to carry around the mistakes you've made, and I couldn't live with this one on my conscience. I needed to get this right. I needed to do the math correctly, I needed to use the staff, and I needed to be assertive, but not aggressive, with the headmistress.

On the tenth breath I envisioned Highspire, the largest building on the academy's sprawling campus and almost certainly the site where they'd focus the evacuation. Since I was wearing my armor I planted the teleport in the sky above the academy so I could do an aerial recon, and then make some decisions.

The staff pulsed in my hand. I could feel Ardaki

watching the situation unfold below, though I had no idea what the weapon thought about it. The idea that a magical item could have a complex intelligence both fascinated and terrified me. Could I talk to it? Could it talk back?

"My gods," I breathed as I took in the sight below me.

Thousands of students had gathered around Highspire, a six-story stepped pyramid at the center of campus that couldn't be more at odds with its name, as it was neither high nor a spire.

Each of the cadets surrounding the pyramid wore a pack and a carried a bedroll. Most had made little camps right where they'd been standing, and there wasn't enough room to lie down, so thousands of azure-robed students leaned against each other, most sleeping, or trying to.

They ranged in age from fourteen to twenty-six, and were divided according to class, with silver- or gold-robed faculty chaperoning them. There were so many. When I'd been a student we never saw everyone lined up, not even during graduation.

"Okay, how to fix this." I peered upwards next, and found a crackling dome of golden energy several meters over my head. As I watched, the ward shrank another meter. "Oh, crap. That can't be good."

That thing must be containing the atmosphere, and was probably stabilizing gravity as well. When it went, the rest of this rock went.

Only then did I realize that I wasn't falling.

I hovered in midair, effortlessly. Was this something the armor was doing? I glanced down at the paper doll. Sure enough there was a violet tinge pulsing from the armor in a sort of aura.

"It must be drawing from the *void* magic," I realized. I hadn't gotten used to having it yet. Thus far, gravity magic seemed a whole lot cooler than having to use thrusters to stay aloft. "Now, about saving these people..."

I thought about drifting lower, and the armor tugged at the new power in my chest. The armor zipped down toward the pyramid, and I started scanning for the headmistress.

She had always been easy to spot, in any crowd. Not because she was tall, or beautiful, or stood out in any way. The headmistress was a short, unassuming human woman with white hair twisted into a bun, and a face like a weathered highway. She was eternal. I had seen my great-grandmother's graduating holopic, and there was headmistress Visala glaring hawkishly at her charges, not a day younger.

No, the headmistress was easy to spot because usually there was a large gap in the crowd around her. No one wanted to be the object of her attention, so students and faculty alike fled as soon as possible.

"There she is." I steeled myself, then zipped toward the top of the pyramid.

The headmistress stood alone at the top of the stairs stretching from the apex of the pyramid all the way to the valley floor. She stared fiercely upwards, but not at me. She was watching the rapidly shrinking ward.

I darted down to her position, and landed more gracefully than I'd have expected. Gravity magic made fine motor control so much easier. So far, having it almost made up for constantly running for my life.

"Headmistress Visala," I called as I willed the mask to slither from my face. Once it had, I introduced myself. "I'm Jerek—"

"Yes, I know who you are, Jerek, son of Dag," she said, her voice a whip, as always. The much shorter woman leaned on a staff of her own, this one a slender golden rod covered up to the midpoint in elaborate sigil work. Unfinished then. "One of my most promising, and least accomplished, students. Average marks. Average attendance. I remember your mother being quite disappointed by your final marks."

"Our world is literally coming apart." I stabbed a finger up at the sky, toward the weakening ward. "How long do we have? An hour? Half that? We need to get these people out. Now. Did the minister brief you?"

I couldn't believe I'd managed all that without breaking and running. I might have sounded like a confident badass, in my own head at least, but it was having an effect. My hands were shaking worse than they had on the tram or after I'd killed the merc.

Visala nodded, then smoothed her robes of office. She turned toward her students, then raised a hand and deftly sketched an *air* sigil, then a *dream*. When she spoke, her voice thundered across the valley and drowned out all conversation.

"Students and faculty," she began, her back firmly in my direction. "I have just been contacted by the minister. She assures me that her people have secured one of the Great Ships for our use. They are going to teleport us into orbit. Gather your things and prepare yourselves as best you are able for our new lives."

Visala made a chopping motion, and the augmentation spell dissolved. She turned back to me, a prim, petty expression on her face. "You *can* live up to what I just promised, yes?"

I glanced around me at the students, and started running numbers. This was going to be close. As a I counted, an awful warbling hum began above, and the ward began to ripple and discolor. This had to be one of the final stages before failure.

"I can." I placed both hands on Ardaki's haft, and concentrated on the weapon. Like me, the staff possessed a connection to the *Word of Xal*, and theoretically I could use its connection to reinforce mine. Instead of casting traditional spells, I merely envisioned what I wanted. Handy, but I still didn't like it, because I couldn't understand why the process worked.

Visala's scandalized voice dragged me back to the present. "Where did you get that staff? It is utterly ancient. It belongs in the armory, and—"

The damage had been done, as I'd known it would be. I'd deal with her knowing about Ardaki later. I tuned her out and focused on my work.

I concentrated on a huge swath of students in front of the temple, nearly a quarter of the total number, and envisioned them teleporting into the designated cargo hold on the *Word of Xal*. I was, as usual, totally unprepared for the results.

The staff slammed down into the temple's steps with so much force it cracked the marble, and earned another scandalized squawk from the headmistress. The dragon's eyes and mouth filled with *void*, and a beam of negative energy that stung my eyes fired into the sky.

The pulse disappeared into orbit, but a moment later an answering pulse came from deep within the glittering fleet, too powerful to ignore even if it produced no visible effect. The students I'd focused on vanished. Every last one of them.

"Sergeant Dag," I said into the comm. "This is Captain Jerek. What's the status report in the hold?"

"Uh, hello, sir," my dad's nervous voice crackled back. "We've had a couple thousand kids appear out of nowhere, just like you said. Are there more coming?"

"A lot more," I promised. "I'll have three more loads just like that one. Make sure the kids don't move from where I teleported them, and keep the center of the room clear at all costs. I don't want them wandering into the other drop points."

"I'll get it done. Good luck, sir."

It was beyond weird having my father call me sir, so surreal that it penetrated the urgency.

"Three more," I muttered. I was still trying to tune out the headmistress, who was staring at Ardaki in a mixture of shock and naked greed.

I focused on the next group of students, and the staff once again fired a *void* pulse. This time, though, it wrenched a huge chunk of power from my chest, and I collapsed to my knees with a cry.

Splitting pain shot through my head, and for an instant every nerve was on fire. It faded quickly, but the dull ache between my temples remained.

I used the staff to haul myself to my feet, and glanced down at the valley. Half the students were gone now. I cleared my throat weekly. "Dad, did you get the second load?"

"Affirmative. Looking good. First group is responding well. Looks like they need a nap."

I gave an exhausted smile, then turned to face the next group. I had to do this two more times, but the thing I most desperately craved in the world was sleep.

A detached part of my mind knew what was happening. The spell was so powerful it was drawing upon my magic, but also my life force. My soul, for lack of a better term. If I pushed too hard...I could die.

I didn't think I was anywhere near that point, though, and I had a job to do. I might not love the headmistress, but

I did love the academy and everything it had done for our world. These kids deserved a future, and by all the gods, dead and alive, I was going to make it happen.

"GrrraaaaaaAAA!!!" I roared as I willed the next group to teleport to the ship. They disappeared, but the backlash was immediate and catastrophic.

I lost vision in one eye as a tidal wave of agony raced through every neuron. I may have briefly lost consciousness, or just been overwhelmed by pain, but when I came to, I was lying on the marble next to the staff.

"Stay with us, mage!" Visala roared. She knelt next to me. "I know it hurts, but you must do this. Just a little more, Jerek. Or, if you cannot manage, give me the staff..."

She stretched out a hand, but moments before it settled on the haft, her flesh dissolved. Two fingers simply ceased to exist, their particles drifting away in a quickly dissolving cloud.

I didn't know what kind of reaction I expected. A scream? Pain? Recoiling? Some physical reaction. There was nothing. Visala stared numbly down at her hand.

After a moment I understood why she wasn't alarmed. Her fingers began to regrow, and within seconds two fresh pink digits had replaced those she'd lost. I could only gawk. Humans couldn't regenerate. What was she?

"It appears," she snapped, her voice icy, "that the staff requires you to complete the spell. You do not have the luxury of failure. Not this time."

"You're right about that." I didn't tune her out. Quite the opposite.

I gave in to the indignant anger. The righteous Jerek who rehearsed speeches in the shower. I channeled every petty revenge thought I'd ever had. Every tough night in the dormitories. Every time a teacher had slighted me, every time I'd been passed over. All of it.

I mattered, damn it, and I was going to show them all.

My hands wrapped around Ardaki's haft, and I willed the last group of students to teleport. More than that. I ordered Highspire itself to teleport. It was only about fifty meters tall, and the cargo bay had about a hundred meters clearance.

I'd save it all, even if it cost my life. Every last book, scale, and student. The armory itself.

The pain was both instant and indescribable. The former waves were gentle touches, a sympathetic reprieve from the agony I had now found. I pushed on with a scream. "I. Will. Do. THIS!"

This time I know I blacked out.

35

I woke up atop the pyramid, and rolled painfully to my knees. Had I failed somehow? No, the terrible humming of the ward was gone. The tearing of rock and endless rumbling of our world tearing itself apart. Gone.

I realized the light was different now. I was still on Highspire, but the pyramid had been moved. I clawed my way to my feet, finally aware of Visala standing near me, her hands clasped primly before her.

Past her were the shining black walls of the cargo bay. I glanced up and saw the cargo bay's black ceiling a good fifty meters over my head. Good thing Highspire's builders hadn't been trying to impress anyone with the height. The whole thing fit snugly.

All around the edges of the cavernous city-sized cargo bay stood groups of students, still organized by class. So many of them. Most were scared, though they were containing it well.

"I can't believe I pulled it off," I muttered as I gaped down at the pyramid and the students. "I saved them all."

"The ship saved them all," Visala corrected. She folded her arms. "You were merely a conduit. I meant what I said about the staff. You need to turn it over for study. It is even more important in light of what has happened to our planet. This ship may be all we have left as a people."

"The staff isn't mine to give. It's on loan, that's all." I turned to face the empty air next to me. "Guardian, you around?"

Kemet appeared with his grin and his illusory staff. I wasn't watching him though. I was watching Visala and her reaction to him. I'd hoped the sight of a magical intelligence this sophisticated would throw her, or distract her maybe.

Her reaction was brief, and lasted no more than a split second, but I was absolutely positive I'd seen what I seen. Recognition. Visala had seen Kemet before, or at least knew of his existence.

"Yes, Captain?" Kemet asked with a bow.

I concentrated on Ardaki's silvered length, and willed the staff back to the center of the core, where it would be safe. Kemet's eyes twinkled and he gave me a fanged grin, though he said nothing, of course.

For a moment I feared Visala was about to make an issue of the staff's disappearance, but she swallowed whatever she'd been about to say and merely watched me, expression neutral.

I focused on the Guardian. "Where is the minister's fleet in relation to us?"

"She is about to dock," he explained. "I have catalogued one hundred and forty vessels in her armada, though only four are capital ships. The smallest is a four-man pleasure yacht."

"Transports and frigates," I muttered. It wasn't a bad thing that they'd survived, but I was hoping we'd have something resembling a navy—though I guess that wasn't my problem. I'd done my part, after all. "Is there a dining chamber or mess where we can receive visiting officers? We want to impress."

"Of course." Kemet nodded, the light glinting realistically off his holographic head. "I would suggest using your own chambers, Captain. They are more than sufficient for a small intimate gathering, and it is the most heavily warded area of the ship."

"I have quarters?" I blinked.

"Captain, you will be taking me with you," Visala demanded, hands on hips now. "I am responsible for these students, who comprise most of our civilization now. I will have a say in what is to come."

A slow half smile grew on my face. "You know what? I think that's a wonderful idea, Headmistress." She might not be an ally, but she'd give the minister something besides me to think about, and I had a feeling that would be to my benefit. "I'm going to use the ship to teleport us to my new chambers. Guardian, can you show me where those are?"

"Of course, Captain." Kemet offered a one-winged bow, much more formal than he'd been previously using. I got the sense he was showing off on my behalf.

An illusory version of the ship appeared next to me, with a blinking green dot over my quarters. There were four rooms. Four! Who needed that much space?

I turned back to Visala and squared my shoulders, ready for battle. A figurative one I hoped. "Are you ready?"

She nodded once, not a hair out of place in that severe white bun. "It isn't my first time teleporting. Let's be about this."

I nodded, then willed the ship to carry us both to "my" quarters.

The main room's opulence seemed out of place on a starship. The bed hovered over the carpet, its pillows still fresh and fluffed despite having been in isolation for countless centuries. It was flanked by two wooden dressers, and not the fake stuff either. The wood was a deep red that reminded me of Shayawood, but darker.

A wide arch opposite the bed led into a sitting chamber, and Visala had already moved through it and found a hoverchair where she made herself comfortable. It matched the chair from the trials, right down to the ghost-tiger fur.

Six chairs bobbed up and down, with a wide table floating in the middle. If they matched what I'd seen of other such furniture, all of it could be adjusted to any desired height. Two of the chairs were larger than the others, probably for hatchlings or similar species.

I moved to the chair opposite Visala, and sat. "Guardian, has the minister come aboard yet?"

"She has, sir," Kemet confirmed. "Shall I direct her to your quarters?"

"Do that," I ordered, "and offer to teleport her if that's more expedient."

"Of course, sir."

We waited in tense silence for several minutes, and then the doors to my quarters opened. There was no knock. Not even a chime. People could apparently just walk in. I'd need to look into whatever security features this place had.

The first pair inside were hard-eyed guards in full spellarmor, though their visors were up, at least, so we could see their faces. The one on the left called over his shoulder. "Clear!"

Minister Ramachan, a woman I'd seen many times on the holo, but never in person, swept into the room. My mother entered a pace behind, and it took everything I had not to run to her like a toddler showing off something he'd found.

"Welcome, Minister," I called, then waved a hand at the hoverchairs. "Please, join us. We're finally getting a chance to catch our breaths."

Ramachan delivered a stately nod as she glided into the room. Her suit was pressed and fresh, despite her probably having been on her feet all day.

"There's much to discuss." She turned back to her guards. "Have the rest of your squad move to protect the bridge, Captain. I'll be heading there when I'm done here."

Resentment surged up in me. She'd only just gotten here and was already making power moves on my ship. The logical part of me knew she was just doing what she had to do, but the rest wished she'd asked me first.

The minister moved to sit in the closest chair, and my mother sat next to her. She gave me a smile, and a little wave, but then it was back to a more professional demeanor.

"Headmistress Visala." The minister nodded at her as she climbed into the hoverchair. "I'm pleased to see you've survived. How are your students?"

She rested her hands in her lap, and adopted a humble expression. "Both my students, and Highspire itself, have been successfully moved. I've yet to examine either, but did verify that nearly everyone made it off."

I noticed that, again, she didn't give me credit for any of it. Had been moved. Not moved by Jerek.

Ramachan must have spotted my expression, because she deftly entered the conversation.

"We're grateful for your assistance, Jerek. You've accomplished the impossible." The minster gave me a practiced smile, though there might have been some genuine warmth there too. She tossed her dark hair over her shoulder, turning to Visala. "I came here tonight with two specific objectives. First, I want to know who did this to our world. We need proof. What do we have?"

That was my cue.

I cleared my throat, and when I had their attention, I spoke. "The head of the Inurans attempting to take control of the *Word of Xal* claimed that he was acting alone, but I believe he was lying. Unfortunately, I had to feed his vessel to the reactor to jumpstart this ship. We weren't able to recover any proof that would directly link this to Matron Jolene."

"Of course not," the minster snapped. Her eyes flashed, and her knuckles whitened on the edge of the chair. "That blasted woman is always three steps ahead of us. She was probably planning this before I was born. I have to believe we will find proof, but I suppose it was too much to expect that she'd left her tracks uncovered. We have a little time until the trade moon arrives, but if we can't find something before then I'm not sure we'll ever find justice."

"The second thing," my mother murmured, just barely audible, but enough to catch the minister's attention. Always the power behind the throne, my mom.

"Ahh, about that." Ramachan fixed me with a stern, but not unfriendly, gaze. "Jerek, I'm going to be straight with you. There's no way we can leave a person with your, ah, record and experience in charge of this ship."

I blinked at her several times, unsure I'd heard her correctly. I licked my lips, and struggled to find something approaching a diplomatic response. I failed. "So let me see if I understand this correctly. I woke a Great Ship, and used it to save Highspire and thousands of cadets while our world literally disintegrated beneath them."

My hand stabbed out toward the wall, almost of its own

accord. I willed that wall to show the space outside the ship, and it obliged. I willed it to focus on our world, and on its final dissolution.

Kemet's last continent-sized chunks were breaking up, and the entire debris field was being pulled into a line as it moved inexorably toward the sun. Our world was done. No one else was making it off.

"Now, after accomplishing that, you think the right move is benching me?" I shook my head. I was angry, and I knew it, but this wasn't fair. Not after everything I'd lived through. "I think you might be a bit more hesitant when you hear what's involved. You want to replace me? Someone needs to don the extra suit of Heka Aten armor we recovered, and then step into the reactor. As the Guardian will tell you... survival is unlikely. Most candidates fail. You want this ship? By all means...take your chances."

The minister cocked her head, then turned to my mother. "I see some of you in him after all."

"Told you so." My mother smiled into her hand.

"I will take that chance," Visala offered. "I'm more than willing to don that armor and bond with the ship."

I knew instantly that the headmistress was after the staff, but couldn't think of a single thing I could say to prevent it. Then I had it.

"Wait," I interrupted. "I have a suggestion. This isn't a decision that needs to be made quickly. I will vacate these quarters, and offer them to the person you name 'Captain'. The ship is almost out of power, and until we solve that, it doesn't matter who you give the title too. I get that I can't run this entire ship, and I don't want to try. But like it or not, I am your only connection currently. Use that connection, until someone on your staff can replace me. Fair enough?"

"And what do you get out of this cooperation?" The minister folded her arms. "I want to hear your price."

"It isn't high," I promised, and meant it. In fact I smiled at her. "I have a small corvette, the *Remora*. I want her and my crew outfitted with all the munitions and supplies we can carry. I want my crew pardoned of any crimes, and I want full autonomy to investigate the Vagrant Fleet. There are other Great Ships out there, Minister, and we need access to them if our people are going to thrive."

The minister was silent for a long time. She never looked away from me, and I struggled to maintain my composure under the weight of that stare.

"Very well," she agreed. Her mouth turned down in a slight frown. "I do not like giving away supplies when they cannot be replaced, but given that you are the only person to take a Great Ship, it makes sense to have you investigate the others. You get your munitions. You get your supplies. I will even pay you. However, you answer directly to me, and I want daily reports."

I didn't like that last part, but she'd given me everything else I asked for. "Done. You've got yourself a relic hunter on retainer, Madam Minister. I know you've got a lot of work to be about. I'll get out of your hair. See you at the next family dinner."

My mother gave a short, amused laugh, which the minister shared. Visala merely glared at me, and I sensed that I'd made an enemy. She knew I was trying to prevent her from getting the staff.

Later. For now I was going to go tell my crew the good news.

EPILOGUE

I strode up the ramp onto the *Remora*, my boots thumping up the now familiar metal. This ship had come to mean so much in such a short period of time. I patted the wall as I entered the cargo hold, unsurprised to see that was where the crew had gathered.

The hold was larger than the mess, with more room to lounge, and since we didn't really have much in the way of food, the mess had nothing to offer other than chairs.

Briff and Rava were laughing in one corner, while my dad hovered nearby, arms folded and his usual dour expression firmly in place. Under that, though, I spied new confidence. His posture was ramrod straight, and he looked around him with pride.

Kurz and Vee stood a few meters away with their matching auburn hair and dour expressions, but more casually, and in less of an attempt to get as far away as possible. I chose to view that as progress.

"All right, team," I called, with as much confidence as I could muster. "I need your attention for about five minutes. Eyes on me."

That got their attention. Once I had it, I wasn't quite sure how to proceed. What if they didn't want to go with me?

"How many of you enjoyed working with the refugees? Raise your hand." I pointedly left my own hand down, and wasn't surprised when no one raised theirs. "Looks like we are all less than excited about it. We're not equipped to run the *Word of Xal*, which now contains a city full of very hungry kids. We *are* qualified to run the *Remora*, though, so I've cut a deal with the minister. We get a full resupply and munitions, and she will even pay us a fair wage."

"To do what, exactly?" my father asked. He shook his head. "It's always a slippery slope with politicians."

I didn't mention that Dad had a specific bias against this one. That wasn't relevant right now. I simply answered the question. "We're going to investigate the Vagrant Fleet. There are other Great Ships out there. Ships we thought past salvage. As it turns out, they masked their drive over-loads, which means that, in theory at least, the other ships could be just as intact as this one."

"We're Relic Hunting?" Rava demanded. She perked up instantly, and leapt to her feet with a whoop. "Are you seri-ous? We get paid to treasure hunt? That is awesome."

"It is pretty much the dream gig," Briff rumbled as he fluffed his wings behind him. "Would we all get an equal share?"

I nodded. "Yes, but captain gets two, and the ship gets one."

"The ship?" Vee asked as she arched an eyebrow.

"We're going to need repairs over time," I pointed out. "If we give the ship a share we'll always have some money to keep it flying. And, if we ever accumulate too much, we can just pay it out to the crew."

"I like the sound of this." Kurz gave an encouraging nod,

and even looked up at me. Briefly. "I am pleased to be a part of your crew, Captain. I have always wanted to explore the Great Ships."

"Well I'm in," my dad added, "so long as my job is fly the ship. I'm good at flying the ship. I don't like leaving the ship. How's that sound?"

"Works for me, but that means we need someone to head up combat ops in the field," I pointed out. "Who do you trust with that?"

"Shit." My dad's scowl came back like a bad rash. "I take it back. I'll be going out in the field. You kids are smart and you learn quick, but you don't have crap for experience and I need to fix that."

"I'd feel better having you in the field," I admitted. I glanced at Vee, who hadn't stated her position. "How about you? Are you in?"

"On one condition, and you know what it is." She removed the band from her ponytail and began retying it. I found myself staring at the curve of her neck. "I won't betrayer the Maker's Covenant, but I will follow any other order you issue, and work to the benefit of this crew."

I nodded. Good enough for me.

"Sounds like everyone is on board except you, Briff. How do you come down?" I folded my arms, and gave the hatchling room to speak.

"Well," he said slowly. "I think I can be an asset to this crew. I've got a lot to learn. My wings are still healing. But if you guys will have me as a heavy, I want this. Like I said, pretty much a dream job. I'm definitely in."

"All right, team. Everyone is on board. We move out tomorrow at 0800. We're done here. Get some rest." I gave them my best lazy salute. "Those of you without quarters, go pick some out."

The room quickly thinned out, but I noticed that Vee stayed behind. She didn't approach me until we were alone, but when she did there was almost a smile. Her lips looked so soft. Yeah, yeah, TMI. I know.

"What's up?" I asked as she joined me.

"You may initiate courtship again, if you wish." She gave an exasperated laugh. "I realize you know very little about my people, and I yours. We are learning, though, and thus far it has been...entertaining. I would enjoy spending more time with you."

Then she turned and rushed from the cargo hold like every Inuran who'd ever owned a rifle was after her. I smiled after her, both surprised and delighted that she seemed interested.

That left me standing alone in *my* cargo hold, on *my* ship. I savored those words.

Against all odds I'd survived the lurkers. I'd survived the dissolution of my planet. I'd survived an Inuran strike team, and a test designed to winnow out all but the best candidates. I'd even gotten paid for it.

But you know what?

I really had to pee.

CAST OF CHARACTERS

Arcan- A heavily cybered merc with scarlet cyber-eyes. Rava's father and the owner of Arcan's Pawn Shop.

Briff- A dragon hatchling with a bit of a gut, and a real love for video games.

Dag- Jerek's father. Former arena champion. Lost his legs during his last op, and now floats around in a hoverchair.

Jerek- Our wise-cracking protagonist. Also an academy trained archeologist with a passion for magical theory.

Jolene- The matron of the Inuran Consortium, one of the most feared organizations in the sector. Mother of Voria, the goddess of light. See *The Magitech Chronicles* for more details.

Guardian Kemet- Dragon hatchling of the *life* dragonflight. The shade of Admiral Kemet, hero of the godswar. Kemet is bonded to the *Word of Xal*, and seeks to guide an officer candidate to become captain.

Kurz- Vee's brother. Kurz is a soulcatcher raised among the lurkers. He is quiet and soft-spoken, but very intelligent.

Minister Ramachan- Ramachan is the 43-year-old leader of Kemet, and is now presiding over the destruction of her world.

Mom (Irala)- Jerek's mother. Former headmistress of the Kemet Academy. Succeeded by Visala.

Rava- Jerek's half sister. Raised by Arcan, but the daughter of Dag.

Valat- The Inuran commander charged with seizing control of the *Word of Xal*.

Headmistress Visala- Visala is ancient, and does not appear to age. Many speculate as to her origins, which are clearly more than human. She is a recent addition to the academy, however, and took over after Irala stepped down six years ago.

Vee- Vee is an enigmatic lurker with vast knowledge of the Vagrant Fleet. Sister to Kurz.

NOTE TO THE READER

If you enjoyed *Dying World*, we have a complete seven-book prequel series with an ending already available, and it leads seamlessly into the book you just read.

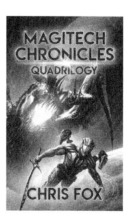

We're also working on a pen & paper RPG and the Kickstarter is going live right around the same time this book came out. You can learn more by signing up to the mailing list, or by visiting magitechchronicles.com and our Magitech Chronicles World Anvil page.

We've got maps, lore, character sheets, and a free set of rules you can use to generate your own character, plus a Facebook group where we geek out about this stuff.

I hope you enjoy and we can't wait to meet you!

-Chris

Printed in Great Britain
by Amazon